Introduction

    I'm no doctor, nor do I have any kind of degree related to the subject matter of this book. As such you are welcome to judge me accordingly but, a whole lot of people have changed the world and the way you live and they did not have degrees either. So I recommend you read this booklet first, before you judge me and I think you will see that a person does not need a degree to be smart, hard working, well informed, and indeed an expert in their field.

    Although the horrendously overpriced rip-off colleges have not put me hundreds of thousands of dollars in debt, I am a consumer and I found myself looking down the massive vitamins and supplements aisle of a typical drug store and realized that there was absolutely no way a person could walk up, pick a multivitamin off the shelf, and get it right.

    Furthermore, I realized that there was no way anyone could pick ANY vitamin or supplement off of that shelf and get it right – that is, try to take something that would shore up what they perceive to be their weakness. And how could a person, like myself, even know what their weakness(es) were in the first place?

    This series of books intends to address this problem. I have done all of the research and I can tell you exactly which products have the best ingredients – which ones work – and where appropriate, which ones have such useless ingredients that they are worth avoiding.

    And that's an important point, it is amazing to consider that some supplements on the very shelf I mentioned are almost completely useless, and it is amazing that they are even allowed to sell the garbage at all, but they are allowed to do it and we all know exactly why: greed and the insatiable thirst to steal that almighty dollar by the millions – the same greed, in the food industry that has made us all sick in the first place!

    If we all stop buying the poisons that the greedy monsters want to shove down our throats, then they will stop wasting their time manufacturing those cancer cocktails and maybe they might actually start making products that are good for us.

    One in three Americans will die of cancer, a disease that was one of the rarest known to medical science prior to World War II with only a handful - and I mean LESS THAN TEN – cases diagnosed by doctors each year. In the fifties these numbers exploded exponentially from hundreds per year to thousands to tens of thousands to hundreds of thousands of new cases each year. What changed? Two things: chemical additives to the foods we eat started appearing in the fifties and the nuclear bombs were set off in the mid forties through the fifties. These bombs create what we all know very well as the mushroom cloud, this thing sends radioactive fallout as high as 30 miles, that's the edge of space, and the upper atmospheric winds can distribute that fallout worldwide and it only takes ONE RADIOACTIVE ATOM to be absorbed by you, to ultimately possibly cause cancer in you.

We have no way of protecting ourselves from the radioactive fallout of these bombs or the Chernobyl and Fukushima disasters that have easily poured ten times the radioactive contamination into the Earth's atmosphere as all of the bombs before them did, but we can stop eating the POISONS that cause cancer and we can start eating the things that will make us healthier.

In this book I have omitted the first chapter on how to identify and stop eating these cancer causing additives to our foods. The only reason I did this is because you can get that information from the preceding book "The Truth About… Vol. 2 – Vitamins" which goes hand in hand with this one anyway. That information is too important to overlook, so I hope you will get the book on Vitamins which are as important and often lacking in our daily diet as well.

I would be remiss if I were to say that clinical trials and studies are the ultimate evidence for proving something: they are not. And I would seem to be a hypocrite if I quoted you one study and said there's the proof and then scoffed at the next study. What I will do is this: I will quote you studies that indicate "No negative outcome." For example, if a study showed that feeding people far more than the RDA of some nutrient had no ill side effects, I will call that "conclusive evidence that the nutrient is safe." I will not quote a study that fed people a metric ton (far more than the normal and usual intake of a particular substance) and that then reported that the substance was toxic. The reason being that too much water is deadly (it is commonly known as drowning,) so these reports are not necessarily of value to us. I will report a study that shows the efficacy of a substance. For example, if a bunch of people are dying of beriberi, and they are given a massive vitamin B complex and return to health, then it stands to good reason that the vitamin B complex worked.

On the other hand I will not quote a study that indicates that something is not effective. The reason for this again is that the study is not necessarily conclusive. For example, giving a massive treatment of a nutrient to people dying of cancer does not mean that the treatment has no usefulness if all of the people died because 1) We do not know what stage of the illness they were in (were they literally on their death beds already?) and 2) We do not know which particular cancer they had; there are roughly twelve major forms of cancer, you know a few of them like benign tumors versus malignant tumors, and tumors caused by a breakdown of the person's autoimmune system versus those caused by exposure to known cancer causing agents and so on. So some things might be highly effective against one kind and have no effect on another, but one thing is for certain: advising a person to stop consuming known toxins and to concentrate on eating healthy foods and taking vitamins, minerals and supplements, while it may not cure carcinomas, won't do any harm either.

I am certain that almost every American who is not actively adding a solid well researched regimen of whole foods or supplements to their diet is MALNOURISHED. Three things are killing Americans:

1. They eat POISON in the form of CANCER CAUSING ADDITIVES to their PROCESSED foods on a DAILY BASIS. (And they are exposed to other POISONS also on a daily basis, like DIESEL ENGINE FUMES, HARSH CLEANER FUMES, etc.)

2. POOR DIET: even if you eat right, most of the plants are being grown in dead soil that has been overused for decades, the only reason the plants grow at all is because of the massive amounts of fertilizers being used on them – artificial, manufactured, chemical concoctions. This is what I affectionately call DIRTOPONICS. Just like HYDROPONICS or AEROPONICS, the plants must be given 100% of their nutritional requirements in order to grow, the only difference is that they are sitting in DEAD SOIL instead of pure water or air while they grow. Because of these conditions, many of the macro- and micro-minerals are dramatically reduced or completely missing, having been absorbed completely out of the soil by crops decades ago. Even the current crops, manage to eek out an existence based on their fertilizer sources of nutrients but cannot possibly be producing the supplements we expect from them in the quantities that they should have, hence we are all malnourished even if we eat the right foods because they simply no longer contain adequate, or natural, levels of the nutrients that they should be providing us.

3. LACK OF EXERCISE: You cannot expect to be healthy if all you do is sit in your car on the way to work. Sit at a desk all day at work, and sit at your TV all evening when you get home. You MUST find a way to do some aerobics, at least one hour DAILY. This series is designed to guide you through the bewildering maze of the vitamin shelf at your favorite drug store and is not a substitute for professional advice. If you are currently on medication of any kind, you MUST CONSULT A DOCTOR before taking anything, including minerals because they STRONGLY AFFECT the way your body works and can actually cause a VERY BAD REACTION in combination with certain strong medications.

Also I have aimed this series primarily at vitamins and minerals but they are ONLY THE BEGINNING, there are a multitude of ESSENTIAL NUTRIENTS that are neither vitamins or minerals. These will be covered here as well.

Now, read and learn.

But the Tomato doesn't have a Nutrition Label, how do I make sure I get my daily recommended dose of vitamins, minerals, and other supplements? The simple answer: you will never know. But I better explain that statement. The FDA's Recommended Daily Allowance or RDA of nutrient "requirements" should say "MINIMUM recommended daily allowance" of REQUIREMENTS since without them you will get sick and die. These values were mostly established back in the first half of the twentieth century with the discoveries of such things as vitamins and so on. For example, the FDA's Recommended Daily Allowance for Vitamin C is 60mg. This might keep you from getting scurvy and dying, but it is nowhere near what a person really needs to stay at the OPTIMUM of health and there is a significant difference between bare minimum survival versus thriving in optimum health or THRIVE-LEVEL amounts of any given essential nutrient.

Everyone knows that Vitamin C can help keep you from catching a cold and it can help you get over one quicker, so we all know that it works with the immune system somehow. Incidentally many "professionals" insist that there is no clinical evidence showing that Vitamin C helps to prevent you from catching colds or from getting sick. This is what I call RIDICULOUS. If one hundred people purposely limit themselves to 60mg of Vitamin C per day I will bet you whatever QUANTITY of MONEY you feel like LOSING that more of them will get a cold of some degree during the next year than another group if they all take 1000mg (or better 2 to 3 thousand mg per day.) And I will bet you all of the MONEY YOU JUST PAID ME from LOSING the previous year's bet that far FEWER of the 60mg/day people will get sick in the subsequent year if they go up to 1000mg/day, so be careful because I plan on taking a LOT OF YOUR MONEY ON THIS BET. And while taking 60mg per day they might not die of scurvy but they will be BARELY SURVIVING and will certainly not be THRIVING and will spend their lives in POOR OVERALL HEALTH until they raise that VITAMIN C daily intake level.

Vitamin C is a "safe" vitamin. And what I mean by that is that you cannot overdose on it (I suppose if you bought a 100 count bottle of 1000mg tablets and took them all in one sitting… you'd probably vomit them all back up and that would serve you right.) It is water soluble, which is part of the reason why you can't overdose on it because your body will eliminate any excess quantity in the urine. Interestingly enough it is highly pungent and easily detected in the urine and I have consumed as many as 3,000mg in a day and my body has never "thrown out" any noticeable excess. Cats make their own Vitamin C, by the way, and those little creatures produce thousands of milligrams of it per day to support those little bodies. We are significantly larger and should therefore need significantly more than they do. Incidentally we lost the ability to make our own Vitamin C when our ancestors discovered that oranges tasted good, and we've been dependent on fruits to get it ever since.

My point here is that most of the recommended minimum daily requirements as posted on those food labels are either ridiculous because they are based on amounts established in experiments conducted over fifty years ago designed to find out where the threshold was between surviving and dying – NOT the threshold of THRIVING and living a LONG and HEALTHY life versus barely hanging on in misery and poor health. Or they are meaningless because they are the average numbers for the herd, and the last time I checked, I am not an average member of the human herd; I do not have 2.4 children, make $30,000 a year, or stand 5'11" tall. And I am very willing to bet that I do not have the same nutritional requirements as average person who has 2.4 children, makes $30,000 a year and stands 5'11" tall either.

So let's take a look at this situation. Here are the FDA's Minimum Daily Requirements for those minerals for which they have established a baseline and bear in mind that there are many nutrients for which they have no idea what the baseline minimum daily requirement for them should be:

Figure 1 - FDA's Minimum RDA Requirements:

Name	A.K.A.s (Forms)	100% RDA
Calcium	Such as Calcium Phosphate	1000mg
Iron		18mg
Phosphorus	Such as Calcium Phosphate	1000mg
Iodine	Iodide or iodate	150mcg
Magnesium		400mg
Zinc		15mg
Selenium		70mcg
Copper		2mg
Manganese		2mg
Chromium		120mcg
Molybdenum		75mcg
Chlorine	Chloride ion	2900mg(1)
Potassium		3200mg
Sodium	Sodium salt ion	2900mg(1)

(1) This seems horribly excessive. The main source is salt, and no one is suffering from "Chloride deficiency" or "Sodium deficiency" by avoiding salt.

It should be noted that there are many more nutrients for which the FDA has not established a Recommended Daily Allowance yet. These include but are certainly not limited to: Boron, Silicon, Vanadium, Nickel, Tin, flavinoids, phytosterols, etc.

NOTE: Nickel is a known irritant and allergen. Be very careful when selecting supplements that contain it.

And we have only just begun! There are nutrients that are still completely undiscovered. How do I know that? Because they are being discovered all the time and no one knows the complete composition and architecture of a single living cell, and humans have trillions upon trillions of them and so do the REAL foods that you eat.

Now some of these supplements are not as safe as Vitamin C. Vitamin A for example is quite dangerous. You can overdose on it and it can mess you up if you do that. This is because it is oil soluble, but not water soluble making it much more difficult to eliminate should you overdose on it and believe me, you can. I did and it is not the kind of experience you want to go through twice, trust me. (I was on medication for severe acne, and one of the programs that I tried was oral and topical Vitamin A combined, my doctor took me off of that within a week when he saw the reaction I had.)

So what we really need to know is which ones are the "safe" ones, that we can pig out on (sort of) and which ones we better take it easy with (bad grammar, ending a sentence with a preposition, I know, but I consider this book a conversation between me and all of my good friends much more than a go for the Pulitzer.) It would also be extremely helpful if we knew what each nutrient offers us so we can pick and choose where we want to pile on heavy and where we might go ahead and stick with the long standing norms listed by the FDA (at least we can be certain that they are not excesses that could cause us trouble.)

That's exactly what this series is all about.

END OF CHAPTER QUIZ
1. The mineral that we need the most of (and which most people do not get nearly enough of) is:
   A.   Calcium
   B.   Phosphorus
   C.   Potassium
   D.   Sodium
   ANSWER: C. Potassium. Humans need at least 3200mg per day, that's three whole grams of it and most people do not get nearly that much..
2. The only nutrients you need to worry about are vitamins and minerals. True or False?
   ANSWER: False. There are many known essential nutrients that are technically not minerals or vitamins. The Omega-3 fatty acids, found in abundance in most fish oils are a good example.
3. The FDA's RDA, Recommended Daily Allowance of any given nutrient:

A. Has been established recently and reflects the latest and most advanced scientific and technological research capabilities of our society.
B. Are always conservative; erring on the side of caution to make sure that any person will always get enough of the nutrient despite differences in weight, height, age, gender, body frame, etc.
C. Have been established for every nutrient your body needs.
D. Were established decades ago and could not take advantage of modern scientific or technological capacities we have now, do not take into account individual differences such as weight, height, build, age, gender, etc, and don't exist for all possible nutrients your body needs, since many of these have not even been discovered yet.

ANSWER: D. The FDA established most of the RDA values back when most people in the U.S. did NOT have indoor plumbing. Think about that. And they are certainly very conservative (just enough to avoid disease) and do not take into consideration an individual's differences and we may never know all possible nutrients that our body needs.

4. Minerals each exist in one form. True of False?
ANSWER: False. This is one of the most confusing things about nutrients; many exist in many different forms and some forms are significantly different from others and we cannot be sure that the form found in nature that is extracted from a natural source is chemically identical to a synthesized one manufactured in a laboratory even if the mad scientists insist that it is.

5. After Calcium and Phosphorus, the next mineral that we need by amount is:
A. Iron
B. Magnesium
C. Zinc
D. Manganese
Answer: B. Magnesium. On average a person needs over 20 TIMES as much magnesium per day as they do iron and most people are not getting nearly enough.

6. The amounts of the minerals are measured in:
A. Ounces
B. Grams
C. Milligrams and micrograms
D. None of the above
Answer: Most minerals regardless of their forms are measured in milligrams (mg or thousandths of a gram) and micrograms (mcg, μg or millionths of a gram.)

CHAPTER 2 – WHAT ARE THE MINERALS ALL FOR?

I'll get straight to it here, but I do want to make a blanket statement concerning all of the following nutrients: whatever it is that we BELIEVE they do for us, it is very likely that they participate much more deeply in the human body than anyone suspects and without them you will indeed die sooner than you should, and you will be miserable and sick all the way to your early and bitter end, so find them and take them. The following chapters will deal with which FORMS ARE THE BEST and which whole natural foods ARE THE BEST ones to eat in order to fulfill your RDA for them..

This listing is set up numbering each major nutrient and then listing their ALTERNATE FORMS below them in the lettered entries below each nutrient.

1. **CALCIUM**: Everybody knows this is the main mineral component in our bones and teeth. However, while the bones do store it and use it as their structural constituent (along with phosphate by the way) the bones do release calcium as needed into the blood stream for other uses that most people are not aware of including: nerve transmission, blood clotting, hormone secretion and muscle contraction. Calcium deficiency can obviously lead to maladies like osteoporosis, but it can also lead to: tooth decay, higher risk of bone fractures, muscle tension, high blood pressure, hardening of the arteries, indigestion, higher risk for heart disease and diabetes as well as certain types of cancer. Calcium rich foods also lead to greater satisfaction after eating which can curb cravings for those on very restrictive diets so Calcium rich foods are a dieter's friend. Calcium is one of the minerals with a very high requirement by the human body and makes up nearly 2% of the average person's total mass. And most foods do not contain enough of it to satisfy our daily requirements and taking straight calcium supplements can lead to serious trouble because we actually need a whole orchestra of nutrients in order to be able to properly absorb it and also use it once it does get absorbed into our bloodstream. Excess raw calcium supplements can and will lead to plaque build up in the arteries which proper intake helps to avoid, and it can also lead to kidney stones which is terrible news.[1]

2. **IRON**: We all know that iron is in hemoglobin in the blood. What you may not be aware of is that it is also in another protein called myoglobin which stores oxygen within the muscle cells and makes it instantly ready to use within the muscle when called upon. While the amount of iron we need each day is not nearly as great as that of calcium, we do need it regularly because our red blood cells don't actually live very long so we are constantly replenishing our red blood cells and constantly

need iron to do that. Currently some experts believe that EIGHTY PERCENT of the world's population are experiencing CHRONIC IRON DEFICIENCY which can lead to some very nasty side effects including: fatigue and weakness, shortness of breath, dizziness, tingling or crawling feeling in the legs, swelling or soreness of the tongue, fast or irregular heartbeat, headaches, poor concentration, depressed immune system, poor digestion including Irritable Bowel Syndrome. Obviously there are symptoms of anemia in this list as expected, and iron deficiency anemia is probably epidemic worldwide if iron deficiency is worldwide. Few foods contain enough iron to meet our daily requirements as well although many foods do contain some iron in them it may not be enough. To make the matter worse, most supplements contain very POOR FORMS like iron oxide a.k.a. RUST which has a very low "biological availability" which means we only absorb about 1% of the iron in the pill when it is in this form. That makes sense because we don't eat rocks, plants do, and only they can use rust in the soil to get their iron with no problem at all.[2]

3. **PHOSPHORUS** – We need about as much phosphorus on a daily basis as we do calcium. Our bones' structures are in fact a complex of calcium phosphate. However phosphorus has a LOT more uses than just bone building. It is found in many amino acids and therefore almost all proteins. It is a primary nutrient requirement of ALL plants and it's the middle number in their fertilizers (i.e. 6-6-6 means 6% Nitrogen, 6% PHOSPHORUS and 6% potassium.) No phosphorus means no protein construction and no new cell growth which leads to death of any organism on Earth. Luckily ALL foods contain large amounts of phosphorus, for the exact same reasons we need a lot of it: it is in all of their cellular structures just like ours.[3]

4. **IODINE** – This one is a BIG DEAL and I am going to go on one of my patented RANTS about this one so hold on to something.

Even the experts are saying that approximately 50% of the world's population may be iodine deficient. And the primary source of iodine in most of the industrialized nations is iodized salt. The problem is that most of these populations have been urged to reduce their salt intake! With everyone avoiding salt, which was the only way to ensure that everyone was getting it in their diet, we are back to square one: iodine deficiency is on the rise again and it can have severe consequences.

Because iodine affects the thyroid gland which is a master gland that controls many other glands within our bodies as well as our metabolism, iodine deficiency can have catastrophic systemic effects on the entire human body. Chronic deficiency can lead to underactive thyroid which tends to slow the metabolism. Low metabolic rate leads to lethargy, inactivity and obesity.

There is little doubt in my mind that our weight problems are coming from our inactive life style based on jobs that involve sitting at computers all day long, but underactive thyroid issues caused by iodine deficiency can definitely exacerbate that situation and encourage a person to be lethargic due to a dramatic drop in their metabolism: we are nation's of obese people because we are suffering from severe chronic iodine deficiency which leads to underactive thyroid, which leads to low metabolism which leads to obesity.

This mineral alone is exactly why I call the "First World" nations of Earth "the best fed and most malnourished populations the world has ever seen."

Iodine deficiency can lead to systemic failures throughout the human body. Chronic shortages lead to the following symptoms: difficulty digesting food, swollen salivary glands and dry mouth, dry skin and/or rashes, poor concentration, short term memory loss, muscle pains and weakness, increased risk of fibrosis and fibromyalgia, increased risk of developmental problems in babies and children, and obviously high risk of thyroid disease such as goiter (extreme swelling of the thyroid gland in the throat.)

The true tragedy of all of this is that it is unnecessary. We do not need a lot of this mineral, in fact too much can also lead to thyroid disease as well. And if a person is convinced that they are not getting enough, a relatively inexpensive supplement can solve the problem.

Excess iodine can be toxic although most people do not get nearly enough and because of this, most experts agree that even though this is possible, it is more important to try to solve the global epidemic of chronic iodine deficiency first and worry about iodine toxicity later.[4]

5. **MAGNESIUM** – Gardeners sure do know about magnesium. It promotes flowering. A shot of Epsom salt around my guava bushes in spring causes them to literally explode in blooms almost overnight. Like most minerals magnesium plays a large number of different roles throughout the human body including but certainly not limited to the synthesis of DNA and the proper utilization of insulin and deficiency is nasty business and has been linked to Alzheimer's disease, diabetes and heart disease to name just a few. While it is in a lot of different foods, it is a challenge to get enough in the daily diet and the World Health Organization estimates that 60% of the adults in the U.S. are not getting enough daily and therefore at risk of disease due to chronic magnesium deficiency. I would call magnesium (and chromium) deficiency the NUMBER ONE CAUSE of DIABETES in the developed nations and it is currently nearly EPIDEMIC in proportion. The main problem with magnesium is

that we do need a lot of it, it is ranked number six in terms of the amount we need on a daily basis. In fact, we need over 20 TIMES MORE MAGNESIUM daily than we do iron.[5]

6. **ZINC** – Zinc has been linked to over ONE HUNDRED enzymatic molecular reactions within the cellular processes of the human body. Chronic zinc deficiency could lead to just about any kind of strange chronic symptoms. Those highest at risk and therefore who need it the most are babies, children, adolescents and pregnant and nursing mothers, Zinc is the essential mineral of the young and growing, but make no mistake about it, adults need it too and it can be a challenge to get enough in our daily eating regimen. Zinc has recently been linked to our immune function and it also serves as a powerful antioxidant and those help our immune system and possibly prevent cancer. And it is currently believed that chronic zinc deficiency is epidemic in the developed nations of the world.[6]

7. **SELENIUM** – This is definitely a micronutrient and our daily requirement is measured in micrograms (millionths of a gram: a lady bug weighs about 1 gram, so our daily requirement would be roughly one lady bug toe nail clipping.) Many healthy foods have enough; the problem is that most Americans do not indulge in these rather specific healthy foods. What is selenium used for in the body? It works with the thyroid just like another weird trace element: iodine. So even if you are getting enough iodine, it won't matter if you don't get enough selenium too![7]

8. **COPPER** – We definitely DO NOT NEED copper which can actually be TOXIC. But we do need a very small amount of it. Sunflower seeds are loaded with all the copper we need. Like most of the metals, copper participates as the "active atom" in some key enzymes throughout the human body.[8]

9. **MANGANESE** – This metal is related to iron and cobalt on the periodic chart of the elements and is chemically very similar and as abundant in the Earth's crust as the other two as well. These three metals have the unusual property that they can change their electronic bonding configuration depending on their surroundings (what atoms come near them) from two bonds to three and then back again. This is very handy and almost ALL LIFE on Earth uses this feature of these metals. (The iron atom in hemoglobin can pick up an oxygen atom in the capillaries in the lungs and then drop it off in another capillary deep in your body because of this.) Manganese is needed in a significant quantity by the human body on a daily basis and is involved in myriad enzymatic functions, but to extreme excess it can be TOXIC because it is so highly reactive and chemically unstable in most usable forms. Manganese is used primarily in proper bone formation and maintenance, wound healing and the absorption of other nutrients. Chronic deficiency can therefore sometimes manifest

itself as any set of symptoms related to other nutrients which are not being absorbed or used properly due to the manganese deficiency.[9]

10. **CHROMIUM** – When we hear this metal's name we think of the wonderful big bumpers of the cars of the 1950's. And those chrome bumpers were indeed plated with this metal. Unfortunately, licking them would probably just make you sick. While chemically quite active, the metal is best absorbed by the digestive tract in biological molecules: best let the plants lick the rocks and the herbivores lick the plants! Chromium plays a vital role in insulin function, brain function, heart function, as well as metabolizing fats, proteins, carbohydrates and other nutrients. Chronic deficiency has been linked to diabetes, heart disease, and neurological disorders. And we do need a significant quantity on a daily basis, enough, that it is likely that chromium deficiency may be the PRIMARY CAUSE of late onset diabetes in the modern world.[10]

11. **MOLYBDENUM** – This is another metal required in very trace amounts, but it is important. It has been found in at least seven different enzymes within the human body and plays a key role in sulfur metabolism. Sulfur is quite common and found in several amino acids. But if we cannot properly metabolize sulfur compounds due to a deficiency in molybdenum, this could lead to liver and brain dysfunction. There have been almost no studies of molybdenum on humans but we do know that it plays a vital role in enzymes in plants. Without it plants will die. And we also know that in extreme excess it can become toxic as well.[11]

12. **POTASSIUM** – This is the one mineral you are likely not getting enough of on a daily basis. It is a critical electrolyte that helps nerve to muscle communication and chronic low levels of potassium can lead to heart disease and heart failure. Most plants are loaded with potassium, but even a vegetarian may not get enough potassium during the course of the day. Low potassium levels are often expressed as muscles spasms including hiccups. And the one muscle you don't want going through spasms is your heart (these are called palpitations and can turn DEADLY in a HURRY.) The system involved is called the SODIUM-POTASSIUM PUMP which moves an electron across a synapse in the nerve to muscle connection. Because BOTH ions are required for this to work we do need to consume BOTH and we need to consume a LOT of them on a daily basis. If you get uncontrollable (unstoppable) hiccups or finger or eyelid twitching, then your body is DESPERATE FOR POTASSIUM.[12]

13. **SULFUR** – This is a macronutrient that is fairly common in all natural foods. It is so common that the FDA has no RDA established for it because they assume that we all get enough

of it. But people who eat very little natural foods could be in trouble. And low molybdenum levels can lead to trouble in absorption or proper utilization of all of that sulfur.
14. **SODIUM** – This is one of the most misunderstood mineral requirements of the human body today. It has been vilified since the late 70's and early 80's as the cause of heart attacks and this is simply NOT TRUE. Without SODIUM and POTASSIUM you WILL HAVE A HEART ATTACK guaranteed. This is because these two ions are what make the nerve to muscle connection work. This electrolytic "pump" is crucial to ALL muscle function and it cannot work without sodium.[13]
15. **CHLORINE** – Normally a TOXIN to all life especially in the forms we are normally exposed to (chlorine fumes released from bleach,) we do need the chloride ion as well for the same reason we need the sodium and the potassium ions, for electrolytic functions and we also need some to make the hydrochloric acid in our stomach. The RDA level is quite high and likely due to the daily loss of chlorine from the stomach down into the rest of the digestive tract although the duodenum is responsible for the reabsorption of hydrochloric acid before it reaches the small intestines where it could burn them.
16. **COBALT** – We know of at least ONE nutrient in the human body that contains this element: Vitamin B12 also known as METHYLCOBALAMIN. It is very likely that we get all of the cobalt we need, if we get enough vitamin B12 in our daily eating regimen and other than that it is likely only needed in very trace amounts if at all. (See Vol.2 – VITAMINS.)

THE REST OF THE MICRONUTRIENTS

There has been very little study concerning BORON, SILICON, VANADIUM, TIN, NICKEL and a host of other minerals that are found in very small trace quantities in the human body. At this time we do not fully understand the roles that they play, but we do know that if they are needed, the amounts are exceedingly small and a healthy diet including fresh vegetables will likely suffice. Boron for example is a trace mineral required by all green plants in order to promote the formation and function of the meristem: the growing tip of a new stem. No boron means no new growth. Since we are 90% vegetarians going back to the dawn of mankind, it is very likely that we have incorporated boron into our bodily needs as well and our vegetables likely bring us all that we need, if we have a healthy natural whole food diet.

END OF CHAPTER QUIZ
1. Which mineral can be TOXIC in excessive quantities?
    A. Molybdenum and manganese
    B. Copper
    C. Iodine

D.   All of the above
ANSWER: D. All of the above. "Megadosing" on minerals is not only unnecessary it can be very dangerous to your health.
2.   Although present in virtually all plant foods, which mineral is the most likely one that people are suffering from chronic deficiency because we need such large quantities of it?
A.   Iodine
B.   Zinc
C.   Potassium
D.   Selenium
Answer: C. Potassium. We are all likely not getting enough of the others too, but potassium which is prevalent in all plant matter, is also needed is very large amounts on a daily basis.
3.   Which of the following currently have no RDA established for them?
A.   Sulfur
B.   Boron
C.   Cobalt
D.   All of the above
Answer: D. All of the above. We do need cobalt in the form of Vitamin B12 which does have a definite RDA established for it, but the mineral itself in any other form does not and it is not known if we need it in any other form at this time.
1.   Which mineral has been linked to proper immune function?
A.   Iron and zinc
B.   Magnesium and chromium
C.   Iodine and selenium
D.   Sodium and potassium
Answer: A. Iron and zinc.
2.   Which minerals have been linked to healthy thyroid function?
A.   Iron and zinc
B.   Magnesium and chromium
C.   Iodine and selenium
D.   Sodium and potassium
Answer: C. Iodine and selenium
3.   Which minerals have been linked to proper insulin function and the maintenance of proper blood sugar levels and usage by the body?
A.   Iron and zinc
B.   Magnesium and chromium
C.   Iodine and selenium
D.   Sodium and potassium
Answer: B. Magnesium and chromium.
4.   Which minerals have been linked to proper synaptic function between the nerve endings and the muscles?
A.   Iron and zinc
B.   Magnesium and chromium
C.   Iodine and selenium

D.   Sodium and potassium
Answer: D. Sodium and potassium
5.   Which mineral in chronic deficiency could lead to kidney stones?
A.   Iron
B.   Zinc
C.   Calcium
D.   Magnesium
Answer: C. Calcium. It can also cause them in excess and without proper additional nutrient support as well.
6.   Which two minerals are so prevalent in plant matter that there is no RDA for one of them because it is assumed that we are getting enough of them?
A.   Iron and zinc
B.   Phosphorus and sulfur
C.   Magnesium and chromium
D.   Sodium and potassium
Answer: B. Phosphorus and sulfur (although phosphorus does have an RDA.)
7.   Fast growing plants like sunflowers and grains likely contain a lot of:
A. Iron
B. Magnesium
C. Iodine
D. Boron
Answer: D. Boron. This is critical to all plants for a functioning meristem for new growth tips of branches and the main stalk. Fast growing plants like sunflowers and grains are loaded with it and often need boron enriched fertilizers. If we do end up needing it (the research is going on now) then sunflower seed kernels, oatmeal and wheat germ will likely give us all we need on a daily basis.
8.   Currently we get our cobalt in:
A. Vitamin B12
B. Methionine
C. Wheat germ
D. No food has cobalt in it
Answer: A. Vitamin B12, or methylcobalamin is named after the fact that it has a cobalt atom in it.
9.   People who avoid all dairy products will most likely have to take mineral supplements in order to get enough:
A. Iron
B. Iodine
C. Vitamin D
D. Calcium
Answer: D. Calcium. Although most dairy products do not contain 100% RDA of Calcium either.

CHAPTER 3 – NATURAL SOURCES OF THE MINERALS

Before anyone goes running break-neck to the pharmacy, they should ALWAYS consider getting their essential nutrients from natural sources FIRST.

If mankind was healthy enough as a hunter-gatherer a million years ago to be able to evolve into the high mental capacity species he is now; then nature does indeed provide us with everything we need. Only in those special cases in which the person has little access to an abundance of fresh foods would they BE FORCED to rely on pills to get the nutrients they need.

It is also fair to assume that our high-intensity agricultural industry has literally stripped the soil bare of all nutrients and we are essentially growing all of that food in dead depleted dust. Because of this the plants rely completely on fertilizers in order to get their nutrients and it is very likely that ALL foods grown in these conditions have far less of the nutrients now than they did a hundred years ago.

CALCIUM

While most carnivores get their calcium from the bones of their prey, digesting bone is not easy even for them and certainly not the best choice for humans either.

But herbivores like cows and rabbits have bones too. So they are getting an ample supply from the plants that they eat but they eat a lot more than we do. As a matter of fact, the calcium in the plants is a much more biologically active and therefore available form of calcium.

It seems strange that plants have lots of calcium in them but they do have it and it should come as no surprise as to what they use it for: structural support of their cell walls. Those calcium compounds sure are tough; almost every living thing on Earth uses them primarily for this function from the plants to the sea snails, to the vertebrates.

Unfortunately we need a LOT of calcium on a daily basis and most plants cannot possibly satisfy our needs for it unless we are willing to eat them all day long like the cows. Luckily, there are several foods high in calcium that we can incorporate into our daily eating regimen that do have high concentrations of calcium; enough to satisfy our daily requirements.

TOP NATURAL SOURCES OF CALCIUM

FOOD	AMT.
1 Cup SARDINES	57%
1 Cup YOGURT	49%
5 oz. CHEESE (most types not processed)	100%

Two cups of yogurt or 5 oz. of cheese each day plus any portion of raw vegetables will cover our need for calcium with natural and healthy forms and this is definitely the way to go rather than choking down chalk pills.[1]

IRON
If 80% of the world's population is suffering from chronic iron deficiency it is a fair bet that YOU are among them. I was and I made sure to straighten that out as soon as I learned that while many foods have it, the average eating regimen of most Americans WILL NOT COVER OUR NEEDS adequately.

TOP SOURCES OF IRON:

FOOD	AMT.
3oz. SPIRULINA	132%
5oz. DARK CHOCOLATE	100%

Given the choice, I will eat Baker's chocolate (pure cacao) dipped in honey rather than a cup of blue-green ALGAE every time. But spirulina, a vegetarian delight, is LOADED with very biologically available iron so you might want to give it a try. Most other foods simply do not have enough to satisfy our daily requirements and this is exactly why MOST PEOPLE on Earth are suffering from chronic iron deficiency. Even beef liver would take 15 ounces per day and I am NOT going to eat a pound of beef liver a day. Thank you very much for the… ahem, "tempting" offer. (It is CRAZY to think that pure 100% dark chocolate has MORE iron in it than beef liver!)

And what about supplements or even iron fortified cereal? Do you know how most iron fortified cereals get their iron? They literally dust the flakes with pure finely powdered iron metal. Don't believe me? Run a magnet through the flakes and see for yourself how it picks up a layer of that iron dust. Now I have no quarrel with feeding our kids pure iron dust. It is absorbable in this form, BUT iron has one nasty feature when exposed to the air: it forms RUST. And a solid brick of iron has very little SURFACE AREA and it still rusts. Finely powdered iron has THOUSANDS of TIMES the SURFACE AREA of a solid brick which means that the powder will turn to rust much faster and RUST has a LOW AVAILABILITY; about 100 TIMES LOWER so we only get about 1% of the iron out of any amount of RUST that we consume. As for iron supplements including MOST of the A to Z vitamins, they provide iron in the form of – you guessed it – iron oxide a.k.a. RUST. Don't waste your time or money on these forms; just choke down the spirulina or ENJOY a big 5 ounce pure 100% cacao chocolate bar dipped in honey. (Not an off the shelf candy bar, they are LOADED with all sorts of nonsense including PROCESSED SUGAR which is all bad for you.)[2]

PHOSPHORUS
All natural foods contain large quantities of phosphorus and a healthy eating regimen of natural whole foods rather than packaged and processed junk will likely cover your needs even though they are quite high (1000mg/day)

Teens can need as much as 4,500mg/day which is ENORMOUS and very difficult to get and might need supplements

to make sure they are getting enough phosphorus on a daily basis.
For the rest of us the solution is simple:
TOP NATURAL SOURCE OF PHOSPHORUS

FOOD		AMT.
1 Cup SUNFLOWER SEEDS	= 1450mg	145%

Sunflower seed kernels are the way to go. If you have read
Vol.2 – Vitamins, then you know they also provide over 100% of
our daily requirements of Vitamins B1, B5 and E as well. They are
a TRUE SUPERFOOD and nothing else in our diet can provide
ALL of the phosphorus we need on a daily basis. An egg for
example provides one tenth of what we need and I am NOT going
to eat ten of them a day. 1 cup of whole milk provides one fifth and
again I am not going to drink milk by the quart (although children
certainly should.) Just get the sunflower seed kernels and be done
with it. They provide SO MANY ESSENTIAL NUTRIENTS that the
body needs that they, and some other superfoods, make covering
ALL of your needs on a daily basis SIMPLE and EASY.[3]
IODINE
My previous rant in the descriptions might not have been strong
enough to impress upon you the importance of getting enough
iodine on a daily basis. And I should stress that getting too much is
also bad for you. You could pop a small potassium iodide pill once
a day, BUT you will be FAR BETTER OFF getting your iodine from
natural sources. They have iodine in much more biologically
available forms and the chances of overdoing it are therefore
much lower as well. (Biologically active or available forms allow for
the easy absorption of the nutrient AND the easy ELIMINATION of
excess amounts as well.)

Because we have heeded the advice of the doctors and
dropped salt from our diets, this is a problem because iodized salt
was how MOST Americans were getting their trace amounts of
iodine each day. So now, without the salt, most Americans are not
getting it and this has led to the epidemic iodine deficiency in most
developed countries worldwide because we rarely if ever eat those
few foods that do have enough iodine in them to keep the thyroid
functioning properly. And underactive thyroid can lead directly to
obesity and I believe this is the PRIMARY CAUSE of obesity in our
country especially in kids. (Being a nation of couch potatoes
certainly helps create the problem, but low metabolism
encourages people to spend their lives sitting around rather than
getting up and out there to do a little exercise – it is all related, one
problem encourages or creates the next one like dominos.)

TOP SOURCES OF IODINE:

FOOD	AMT.
SEAWEED (like kelp)	From 10% to 2000%
5 oz. COD (wild caught)	>100%
2 cups organic YOGURT	≈100%
½ teaspoon of IODIZED SALT	≈100%

Seaweed is quite variable as to how much iodine it could contain and iodine deficiency is lowest in countries like Japan where seaweed is definitely on the menu. While I do love cod and have it on occasion it is not something that I can eat daily and that leaves the yogurt. Organic (grass-fed cows) yogurt is loaded with iodine as well as many other essential nutrients and I recommend 2 cups per day because this too makes getting ALL of your daily nutrient requirements SIMPLE and EASY.

For those who have no other recourse, do yourself a favor and make sure you put at least ½ teaspoon of IODIZED SALT in something you cook during the day and make sure that you eat ALL of the food in that pot including the liquid (something like soup is perfect.) That will cover your need for iodine.[4]

MAGNESIUM

Here is another mineral that most people are likely not getting in sufficient quantities that their bodies need. While it is present in most plant foods (it is the "active ingredient" in chlorophyll,) it may not be enough to satisfy our daily requirements unless we eat those plants by the bushel.

TOP SOURCES OF MAGNESIUM:

FOOD	AMT.
1 cup SPINACH (cooked)	≈40%
5 oz. DARK CHOCOLATE	≈100%

I don't usually eat 2.5 cups of spinach per day, though I do eat about ½ to 1 cup raw for the vitamin K. About the only food on Earth that has enough magnesium in it to be practical to eat on a daily basis is DARK CHOCOLATE! So I am really not kidding when I highly recommend it. It is the most practical way to get all of the IRON and MAGNESIUM your body needs. Just make sure that it is PURE 100% CACAO and NOT some processed junk with flavoring and other nonsense in it. It is the TRUE CACAO that contains all of the rich essential nutrients that we need. And it is very bitter which is why I dip it in honey. If you are starting to learn how I operate then you know that I dip it in honey for a REASON: Honey is a powerful natural curative/preventative food too.[5]

ZINC

This is another essential mineral wrapped up in a lot of enzymatic function throughout the entire human body that most people are not getting in sufficient quantities on a daily basis. Zinc is also suspected of playing a key role in our immune system and chronic deficiency could lead to susceptibility to colds and flu as well as far more sinister problems later in life like cancer.

Unfortunately there is no single SUPERFOOD source of zinc and you might have to find a GOOD supplement to make sure you are getting enough of this vital essential nutrient.

TOP SOURCES OF ZINC:

FOOD	AMT.
7 oz. of LAMB	≈100%

1 cup PUMPKIN SEEDS   ≈45%
9 oz. BEEF (organic, grass-fed)   ≈90%

I will gladly sit down to a nice big steak, but I personally can't afford to do that every single day and two cups of pumpkin seeds is a bit excessive and my local grocery store does not carry lamb at all and I wouldn't know how to prepare it anyway. But if you can get lamb meat then I highly encourage you to do so. It is loaded with vitamins and minerals that your body needs and can help you knock out your RDA needs for MANY essential nutrients for the day.[6]

SELENIUM

Luckily we do not need very much of this mineral, but unfortunately it is not found in very many foods in the quantities that we need despite those microscopic amounts that are required. Selenium is also needed by the thyroid for proper function and I suspect that a shortage of selenium in our daily diet is just as likely the cause of epidemic underactive thyroid and obesity as a shortage of iodine.

The average adult is said to need about 70mcg (micrograms) which is indeed a tiny amount, but most foods contain so little that we can't even get that tiny amount out of them on a daily basis. Luckily there are a few SUPERFOODS LOADED with it.

TOP SOURCES OF SELENIUM:

FOOD	AMT.
BRAZIL NUTS (two whole)	>100%
SUNFLOWER SEEDS (1 cup)	>100%
SARDINES (5 oz.)	≈100%

Just TWO Brazil nuts contain your daily requirement of selenium. They are literally LOADED with it. I chop a bunch up into my trail mix and snack on that daily but the majority bulk of my trail mix you might have guessed is SUNFLOWER SEEDS, and 1 cup of them will fulfill your daily requirement of this essential nutrient as well. I cannot possibly stress enough, how GOOD sunflower seed kernels are for you. That goes for sardines as well. And I do eat them on occasion, but certainly not daily.[7]

COPPER

This is an unusual essential nutrient because it is definitely DANGEROUS in excess. However, we do need it and it is involved in several energy related enzymes in the human body.

TOP SOURCES OF COPPER:

FOOD	AMT.
Beef liver (1 oz. organic)	200%
Dark chocolate (5 oz.)	≈50%
Chick peas (Garbanzos; (1 cup)	≈30%
Lentils (1 cup)	≈25%
Sunflower seed kernels (1 cup)	≈25%

The sunflower seeds and the dark chocolate currently resolve most of my personal need for copper and most of the rest of the natural foods that we eat have much lower quantities. As such it is very likely that most folks are getting SOME copper but not enough to meet their THRIVE-LEVEL requirements. While extreme excesses of copper can be toxic, I suspect that natural whole food sources are far less likely to reach toxic levels when compared to artificial inorganic forms found in most supplements. To underscore the point, a lot of people are eating a lot of beef liver and a 3oz portion contains 600% of the RDA and they are not getting copper poisoning.[8]

MANGANESE

Manganese is a very chemically active metal and while it is essential to all life and can be found in fresh vegetables, excesses of it can be TOXIC. You will likely never suffer from excesses though because there are few SUPERFOODS loaded with it because excesses are usually TOXIC to ALL LIFE.

TOP SOURCES OF MANGANESE:

FOOD	AMT.
3 oz. MUSSELS	≈250%
3 oz. CLAMS	≈250%
1 oz. WHEAT GERM	≈250%

After these sources the amounts fall off sharply and usually require you to eat far too much of the food to be practical: However, the real winner here is the wheat germ which is the little nugget of nutrients within the wheat seed that the little wheat embryo will grow on first to swell and get out of the seed shell. Wheat germ is LOADED with many essential nutrients and for this reason it is a SUPERFOOD and I highly recommend it. I dump about a 1/4 cup into my oatmeal which I have three or four times a week for breakfast. That will definitely cover my body's need for manganese! Remember that in this form it is in a biologically active and available form which the body can take in easily and also discard what it doesn't want with equal ease. Taking supplements you might be getting it as an oxide (manganese RUST) which has a much lower availability and that is a form much more likely to cause manganese TOXICITY in the human body as well. I never heard of anyone suffering from manganese poisoning up in Maine from eating too many clams so go for it![9]

CHROMIUM

This is possibly number three on my list of essential minerals that most people are simply not getting enough of over long periods of time which can and will lead to terrible health including but not limited to DIABETES. (Iron and potassium deficiency are number one and two, by the way.)

Because chromium is so critical to good health and the maintenance of proper blood sugar levels and assists insulin you cannot afford to scrimp on it and the medical industry is not entirely convinced that manufactured supplements are both safe and effective, To that end, it is very important to make sure that you are getting enough from natural food sources.

TOP SOURCES OF CHROMIUM:

FOOD	AMT.
1 cup BROCCOLI	≈88%
1 cup GRAPE JUICE (pure, unsweetened)	≈32%
1 teaspoon GARLIC	≈12%

Although I can't find the numbers for raisins, which are simply dried grapes, I am sure that they are LOADED with chromium as well (it certainly won't evaporate.) I included the garlic because I cook with it DAILY and HEAVILY. Garlic has TREMENDOUS nutritional and curative/preventative properties as well. I do not eat broccoli daily, though it is definitely on the menu as an excellent plant source of biologically available CALCIUM as well as CHROMIUM. But I do drink WELCH"S 100% PURE AND NATURAL CONCORD GRAPE JUICE in large quantities DAILY to take care of TWO separate needs: 1) Chromium, and 2) It contains an active substance that very literally DISSOLVES ARTERIAL PLAQUE very slowly and very safely. It is the natural substance that was discovered in CONCORD grapes that inspired the creation of the "roto-rooter" drug given to stroke and arteriosclerosis patients to help clear blood vessel blockages of heavy plaque build up.[10]

Many people do not like the taste and I don't care for it much myself so I mix it half and half with ALOE VERA JUICE as well. ALOE is one of the most powerful and amazing of all of nature's bounty and many doctors worldwide are convinced that it not only cures many chronic digestive maladies but that it also CURES CANCER especially digestive tract forms.

Now I am no doctor and the reports may well be no more than anecdotal at best and if you have cancer of any kind you MUST see a doctor and follow their plan to treat you, but that doesn't mean that ALOE doesn't work either. Just mention it to your doctor that YOU WILL BE DRINKING IT IN LARGE QUANTITIES DAILY whether they like it or not.

MOLYBDENUM

This is another mineral that we require in very small amounts and that can definitely reach toxic levels in excess. Fortunately, even though all plants need it, they too only have trace amounts normally available to them as well.

TOP SOURCES OF MOLYBDENUM

FOOD	AMT.
230 cal. LENTILS	≈330%
230 cal. GREEN PEAS	≈300%
230 cal. OATS	≈100%

So now you know exactly why I include oatmeal as one of my regular breakfast meals at least three to four times a week. Lentils and green peas are also very nutritious and I highly recommend them as well even though they are technically speaking SECONDARY FOOD sources. Anything that needs to be cooked in order to become edible is a secondary food source that should be REDUCED to being eaten sparingly and only on rare occasion. Lentils, green peas, chick peas and oatmeal are the exceptions to this rule because they are loaded with excellent essential nutrients.[11]

POTASSIUM

Here we go – this is the BIG ONE. Even though potassium is prevalent in most plant matter, it is still usually not enough to satisfy our HUGE DAILY REQUIREMENT of it. Cooking plant matter is a problem because potassium is highly soluble too so boiling vegetables quickly depletes them of potassium which is exactly why I recommend eating as much RAW vegetable plant foods and fruits as you can on a daily basis.

While bananas are renowned for being high in potassium, they DO NOT COME CLOSE to satisfying our daily intake requirements. One large banana holds about 14% of our daily requirement and I usually do not eat SEVEN to EIGHT of them per day which is what you would need. They are good and they do have some potassium in them as well as dopamine which is a mood enhancer, so they should definitely be on the menu for everyone, but DO NOT THINK that eating anything short of a huge bunch will satisfy your RDA requirements of potassium.

Chronic potassium deficiency is EXTREMELY DANGEROUS and can lead to SUDDEN ACUTE DEFICIENCY which CAN BE DEADLY. Potassium and sodium function within the synapses between the nerve endings and the muscle cells and if they fall to critical low levels you can get those bothersome uncontrollable muscle twitches that I used to get in my little finger and eyelids all of the time. But sudden acute drops in potassium could deplete the heart muscles of this important linkage to the nerves and BANG: heart palpitations (uncontrolled twitching like your finger tip or hiccups) and DEATH from a heart attack.

Once I shored up my daily potassium intake those irritating twitching sessions in my fingertips and eyelids, as well as frequent heavy and intolerable bouts of hiccups magically vanished. I can't remember suffering from any of that for YEARS.

If bananas are very HIGH in potassium yet still fall way short of our daily requirements you can bet that getting enough daily is a bit of a hassle, but there is ONE SOURCE that will take care of your needs quickly and easily: Low Sodium Vegetable juice. They load it up with potassium salt to maintain the salty flavor. So much so that 24 oz. will cover 70% of your requirement of potassium.

TOP SOURCES OF POTASSIUM

FOOD	AMT.
1 large AVOCADO	≈30%
≈24 oz. LOW SODIUM VEGETABLE JUICE	≈71%
1 large BANANA	≈14%

While I do love avocados, I am not about to eat THREE of them a day, and that is about the BEST natural food source of potassium on Earth. You can tell that I am purposely trying to avoid mentioning a name brand but this nutrient is simply too important to leave to chance: Buy LOW SODIUM V-8 and read the label and drink enough of it to cover at least 70% of the RDA requirement of potassium every day and you will NEVER have to worry about this extremely important nutrient ever again. But don't neglect the bananas either: 2 a day are still excellent snacks that help you reach 100% RDA and they are far better than those DEADLY packaged junk foods.[12]

SULFUR

Sulfur is the stinky nutrient and it is easy to recognize because of this. Ever wonder what makes skunks clear the room? They give off a sulfur compound that is purposely noxious to the extreme, and sulfur rich foods are equally odiferous although I happen to love their aromas (skunks no, but garlic yes!)

There is no RDA value assigned to sulfur because the assumption is that most people on a healthy nutritious diet get enough, but that is not necessarily true. If you do convert your daily eating regimen from one filled with packaged processed garbage food and start eating all natural whole foods then you are well on your way to converting your daily diet from one loaded with artificial CANCER CAUSING CHEMICAL COCKTAILS and TRASH calories from things like partially hydrogenated soybean oil and high fructose corn syrup to one loaded with essential nutrients and high quality calories, but just to be on the safe side I like to include sulfur rich foods in my daily regimen as well.

TOP SOURCES OF SULFUR:

EGGS

GARLIC

BROCCOLI and CAULIFLOWER

SODIUM

High sodium is a definite problem and we have gotten the message; most people are cutting way back on salt in their diets and that is a good thing. But we do still need sodium in our diet because sodium and potassium form a "Sodium-Potassium pump" in the synapses between the nerve ending and the muscle cells that allows the nerves to control those muscles and when the body's levels fall too low, those synapses start to fail and that can be disastrous since the failure of ONE particular muscle – your heart – can cause DEATH rather quickly.

It is truly ironic that the medical industry clamored for us to reduce our sodium in order to reduce our risk of heart attack, but the ion is still required and in surprisingly HUGE AMOUNTS on a daily basis.

Regular exercise and proper levels of potassium on a daily basis as well as drinking plenty of fluids including ample amounts of water virtually ELIMIINATES the potential threat posed by sodium. And because IODIZED SALT is just about the ONLY WAY most people are going to get that critical IODINE, then I do highly recommend that you cook with about 1 teaspoon of IODIZED SALT each day. That will more than cover your needs for BOTH IODINE and SODIUM. No need to go overboard with it and that is what was causing the problem 30 years ago when the medical industry went on their anti-salt crusade.[13]

CHLORINE

I have never heard of anyone suffering chlorine deficiency, but it does play a vital role in certain ionic receptors in nerve endings and we do need a little to replenish the hydrochloric acid levels in our stomachs. The same 1 tsp of IODIZED SALT in our food on a daily basis will likely supply us with all of the chlorine we need.

COBALT and the OTHER TRACE MINERALS

Cobalt is a key component of the Vitamin B12 molecule and for now, as far as we know, that is the only place we need it. Vitamin B12 is critical to healthy brain function and I cover this all-important nutrient in Vol. 2 – Vitamins. As for the rest, they are all under investigation and their roles in the human body are yet to be fully understood. Suffice it to say that as long as you are eating a healthy diet of natural whole foods and eliminate packaged processed garbage foods from your diet you will probably be getting a lot of these trace nutrients that our bodies need – even if we don't yet know why!

END OF CHAPTER QUIZ

1. Which of the following has the highest number of people experiencing chronic deficiency?
   A. Zinc
   B. Iron
   C. Iodine
   D. Cobalt
   Answer: B. Iron. The World Health Organization estimates that up to 80% of the Earth's population are not getting enough iron on a daily basis.

2. Which of the following is the most difficult to get in sufficient amounts on a daily basis (no true superfoods loaded with it)?
   A. Zinc
   B. Iron
   C. Iodine
   D. Cobalt
   Answer: A. Zinc. One of the best sources is pumpkin seeds but it will take 2 cups daily to meet our requirements.

3. Which mineral is the active atom in a vitamin and we likely get all we need if we get enough of that vitamin?
   A. Zinc
   B. Iron

C. Iodine
D. Cobalt
Answer: D. Cobalt. The mineral is the active atom in Vitamin B12 and like most of the other trace minerals, cobalt is currently under study.
4. Which mineral is mostly found in seafood?
    A. Zinc
    B. Iron
    C. Iodine
    D. Cobalt
Answer: C. Iodine. Some forms of seaweed are loaded with it but it is also found in most oceanic fish and shell fish as well.
5. The very best natural source of Selenium is:
    A. Brazil nuts
    B. Sunflower seeds
    C. Sardines
    D. All of the above.
Answer: A. Brazil nuts. It is found in sunflower seeds and sardines as well, but Brazil nuts have the highest concentration of any food and are the very best source.
6. The most practical source of Manganese is:
    A. Mussels
    B. Clams
    C. Wheat germ
    D. Sardines
Answer: D. Wheat germ. This is available in most grocery stores and you don't need a lot to get your daily fill. Oceanic shell fish are literally loaded to the gills with it as well.
7. Which food is high in sulfur?
    A. Fish
    B. Sunflower seeds
    C. Beef liver
    D. Eggs
Answer: D. Eggs. Most stinky foods are very high in sulfur including fish, broccoli, and garlic as well.
8. Aside from iron what is the next most likely mineral with an extremely high chronic deficiency rate worldwide because we need so much of it daily?
    A. Calcium
    B. Magnesium
    C. Potassium
    D. All of the above
Answer D. All of the above are needed in relatively large quantities by the human body on a daily basis and it is a real challenge to find whole natural foods that will satisfy those daily requirements of them. Potassium is found in virtually all natural foods, but we need a lot; so much that even high concentration foods like bananas are simply not good enough.

CHAPTER 4 – THE GOOD, THE BAD, AND THE UGLY
MINERAL SUPPLEMENTS ON THE MARKET

Again, I am not really here to bash any particular name brand of product, and taking anything, even rocks, is better than not taking anything at all, but while you night absorb 1% of the rock dust you are taking as one of the minerals in the form of its oxide, you will do much better taking the mineral in a form where you absorb MOST of what you bought. These supplements are not cheap and to pay $10 for a bottle, only to actually absorb 1% means that you will be getting 10 CENTS of what you paid for and be sending the other $9.90 cents of it right down the drain.

Remember the absorbability, solubility, and "biologically active" forms when shopping.

TIPS: Don't buy a supplement if the company cannot be found on the Internet, and does not provide you with a land address and phone number which should be in the United States. (The government gets touchy about us buying things like this from another country.) Check the manufacturer out at the BBB. And why not? If they are providing ineffective products or poisoning people with them, you ought to know right? A word on the BBB site: a company with a lot of sales will have a lot of complaints just because Americans like to whine and bellyache about every little thing and try to get everything for free – that is if they can't find a way to sue outright, which has gotten to the point that quite frankly makes me sick, but be that as it may, you want to look at percentages of customers that are upset. Small companies with one or two or a few situations is OK, but a couple had dozens of problems and these are low volume businesses, so I avoided them – you get the idea.

NATURAL SOURCE NUTRIENT SUPPLEMENTS

Any time you can find a vendor selling minerals extracted from natural sources, these will be the very best ones and admittedly they will be more expensive than the artificially manufactured ones. However, I personally would rather go without, than to consume artificially manufactured chemicals of any kind ESPECIALLY minerals and other essential nutrients. If I am willing to PAY for these products it makes sense that I should be willing to pay for things that will make me healthy – not things that could very likely make me sick or even KILL me.

Obviously, your number one source of all of your minerals and essential nutrients should be the food that you eat on a daily basis, but it is very difficult to find some of those nutrients in sufficient quantities in natural foods that we would also be willing to eat in sufficient quantities on a daily basis. For example, 5 oz. of pure 100% cacao dark chocolate provides 100% of the RDA of magnesium (and iron) and I do eat this most days. However, if I couldn't find a supplement containing CHELATED MAGNESIUM – a form in which the magnesium is in an organic molecule – then I WOULD EAT 5 OUNCES OF PURE DARK CHOCOLATE EVERY DAY. That is, magnesium is wrapped up in far too many processes throughout the body to risk coming up short on it and FAKE manufactured magnesium in inorganic mineral form is completely UNACCEPTABLE. I would gladly eat the bitter chocolate slathered in honey before eating that potentially DANGEROUS and definitely INEFFECTIVE manmade garbage. You have been warned.

MULTIVITAMINS

Virtually all of these "A to Z" supplements have a LOT of ingredients that are in UNUSABLE forms: this means that our digestive tracts cannot get the nutrients out of them in the forms they are putting in the pills. An excellent example of this is iron in the form of ferrous oxide a.k.a. RUST. We cannot digest this and only get about 1% of the iron out of the amount they are putting in the pill even though the nutrient label indicates that the pill contains 100% of the RDA of iron. This is by WEIGHT and the iron is in there in the amount they say, but our digestive tracts cannot get it out of those RUST molecules and it passes right through you and you get almost nothing from it.

And most of the rest of the ingredients are manufactured FAKE, SYNTHETIC, MANMADE GARBAGE versions of the minerals as well. For minerals like magnesium that we need in large quantities we cannot rely on manufactured inorganic mineral compounds like magnesium sulfate to be able to provide the correct amount in a SAFE and USABLE form. In this case, it would yield the bare lone magnesium ion which happens to be a potential problem in excess. Any metal ion in excess could lead to metal poisoning, even those that we need and can absorb as lone ions.

Although it is a bit more trouble to have to chase down each essential nutrient one at a time and purchase them in natural source forms or at the very least organic molecular compounds, and be forced to take a bowl full of pills before each meal, if they are GOOD versions of the ingredients – "biologically active" or "absorbable" – then these are SO MUCH BETTER for you, and you GET ALL OF THE PRODUCT you are paying for, that they really are worth the extra effort.

Sometimes I coordinate which ones I am taking with my daily food regimen as well. If I plan to eat 5 ounces of dark chocolate then I do not have to take an iron or a magnesium supplement.

This is a critical consideration concerning copper and several other minerals that can be toxic in excessive quantities. If I am going to eat a 1 cup of sunflower seeds (loaded with copper) then I should NOT also take my copper supplement for the day. Remember that extreme excesses of copper COULD be toxic and the best defense for that is 1) to maintain a very healthy and complete essential nutrient daily intake regimen (all of the essential nutrients play very complicated roles throughout the human body and the deficiency of any ONE of them could have a drastic effect on how the other ones are absorbed or used by the body) and 2) Try to get ALL of those essential nutrients in their natural whole food sources. We know practically NOTHING about the gigantic complex array of molecules in these natural whole foods and the roles they play in the digestive tract as well as which ones are absorbed and how they interact with the essential nutrients throughout he body in supportive and possibly very critical roles with them within the cells as well.

So this coordination takes a little effort and a little time. I would rather pay attention to what is going into my body and make sure it is GOOD and SAFE and in PROPER AMOUNTS, than waste that time watching some moronic sitcom on the boob tube. That millionaire comedian only cares about ratings and the big fat paycheck from the executive producers. I prefer to spend the time making sure I OUTLIVE HIM so I can get the LAST LAUGH.

PRODUCTS TO AVOID

Obviously any pills containing artificial colors, flavors or preservatives and this would include most children's chewable vitamins unless they specifically state that they are NOT putting those things into the product or you read the label and don't see them in there. (See the first chapter of Vol. 2 – Vitamins for the details on identifying artificial chemicals in your food products and yes, they do put them in supplements, especially chewables.)

When it comes to the minerals, especially the metals, most OTC (Over The Counter) products on the shelves of the big stores are loaded with INERT, UNAVAILABLE, INORGANIC forms and are largely ignored by the digestive system and pass right through us like the aforementioned RUST pills claiming to contain 100% of the RDA of iron. They do by weight but NOT by the amount you actually absorb from them.

CALCIUM

Calcium is a HUGE nuisance in MOST products because it is provided in the form of either CHALK, PLASTER OF PARIS or CONCRETE (Calcium carbonate, calcium sulfate, or calcium phosphate) and while we can get the calcium out of these products it is NOT IDEAL AT ALL. Even dogs have trouble digesting crunched up bones and humans CERTAINLY have problems with things like that.

Rather than choke down horse pills of chalk or plaster-of-Paris, you should look for "biologically active" or "available" forms. The number one reason for this is that these are far easier for our intestines to absorb and for our livers to handle. Don't forget that every molecule you eat that gets taken up by the intestines passes through the liver to be sorted and warehoused until the liver decides it is needed and then releases it into the bloodstream including calcium and every other mineral. Some things can be released as simple naked ions, but others have to be wrapped up into an organic molecule in order to be transported safely through the blood: the easier it is for the liver to do the chemistry on what you ate, the better.

It is also critical to remember, especially for those taking calcium to avoid osteoporosis and other bone degenerative diseases, is that the bones also warehouse calcium and will release it back into the blood when it is needed by other systems in the human body; that is part of their job. Knowing that calcium is NOT JUST for bones and teeth, but other biochemical systems in the body need it as well and will deplete the bones if it is not being taken up in sufficient quantities in our daily diet, means that we must strive to make sure that it is in our daily diet.

The very best sources are dairy products and the highest concentration of biologically available calcium is yogurt (2 cups a day) or any unprocessed cheese (5 oz.) will fulfill your daily requirement and STOP the erosion of the bones caused by OTHER systems in your body demanding it. If it is there already in your daily eating habits then the liver can release it in to the blood stream without the bones having to give it up.

Megadosing on calcium especially inorganic forms can be dangerous for two reasons: 1) It can lead to kidney stones which are, from what everyone who has had them tells me, not fun, 2) there is MORE to calcium than simply taking a truckload of it. Excess calcium WITHOUT a proper amount of Vitamin D3 also present means that the calcium cannot be properly utilized by ANY system, especially the bones. So where will all of that calcium go? It will form plaque on arterial walls and stones in your kidneys. And the story doesn't end with Vitamin D either. You also need appropriate levels of Magnesium and vitamin K to make sure that the calcium is being properly handled in the body.

As such you should stay near the RDA of calcium and also be very sure that you are getting ample amounts of magnesium, Vitamin D and vitamin K and all of these should be coming from a proper natural whole food source diet rather than pills. Messing with the delicate and complicated system of calcium will definitely do more harm than good.

CORRECT FORMS

If you cannot for some reason eat 2 cups of yogurt or 5 oz. of natural cheese (any kind will do) each day (perhaps you are lactose intolerant) and are forced to take a supplement, then the best form that I have seen on the market is Calcium citrate. The calcium is bonded to citric acid or the citrate ion which comes from citric acid when reacted with something like calcium hydroxide. So the calcium is in an organic molecule and is very highly likely in a usable and available form that does not cause nearly the trouble that the inorganic rock forms do. Just be sure to also take magnesium and natural vitamin D3 AND natural vitamin K1 OR K2 to complement all of that calcium you are taking. Oh, and drink LOTS of WATER (to help the kidneys if too much starts showing up in the blood and the kidneys are forced to remove it.) Oh, and while you are taking all of that vitamin K you better complement that with a good supply of NATURAL vitamin E to prevent internal blood clotting which could be caused by the sudden hike in vitamin K. So now this has snowballed all the way into the need for an oil soluble vitamin (E) that cannot be megadosed. So you must stay CLOSE to the RDA's for all of these nutrients. If you are just taking calcium as a preventative, you do not have to overdo it. Most people get osteoporosis and other such bone maladies late in life due to long term chronic calcium deficiencies over periods of decades. As long as you get the right amount daily in a usable natural form and balance this with the helper nutrients, you should be able to avoid those problems in the future.

IRON

Almost ALL of the OTC products are RUST or some other mineral similar to RUST that are UNAVAILABLE FORMS. The number one most effective form is "Heme iron" which means it is made from animal blood like red beef meat. This goes all the way back to our deep dark evolutionary past when we used our canine teeth and before we mastered fire. I am not advocating blood pudding, or eating a giant steak every day, just stating a fact.

Plant iron like that found in spirulina or dark pure 100% chocolate is a close second when it comes to the best possible form of iron to take. And these are the only two natural foods that are loaded up with a high enough concentration of iron to be able to eat reasonable quantities daily and satisfy our rather large iron requirements.

GOOD FORMS

If you can't stand the taste of spirulina and are allergic to chocolate, then you will likely be forced to take a supplement. Try to find a natural source iron supplement before you try others like iron fumarate (an organic molecule, but it is manufactured and we do not know how effective or safe it is in this form.)

PHOSPHORUS

By far the highest concentration of phosphorus in just about any food is found in sunflower seeds. Do yourself a favor and eat at least ½ cup of the kernels each day. This will provide you with roughly 100% RDA of: Vitamin B1, B5, E, Phosphorus and Selenium. One food just knocked out FIVE of your FULL daily nutrient requirements: Sunflower seeds are the TOP nutrient dense SUPERFOOD on planet Earth; nothing else provides so much in such a small amount.

All other choices are not nearly as dense with phosphorus and would force you to eat them by the bushel. Since phosphorus is a macronutrient used in the construction of several amino acids which means it ends up in all of our proteins and even our DNA, as well as the bones and teeth, an inadequate supply (and we do need a LOT of it on a daily basis) will slow cellular division and new cell formation which slows the turn around regeneration of ALL organs and systems in the human body. This leads to premature aging and the degeneration of ALL organs and systems in the human body as well. And this can be solved with one little handful of sunflower seed kernels.

GOOD FORMS

Phosphorus is generally found in OTC supplements in the form of the phosphate ion (like calcium phosphate which is basically concrete) and these mineral or inorganic forms are the worst forms you could take. Since the primary use of phosphorus is the synthesis of amino acids why bother eating concrete? Just get the phosphorus in amino acids (complete animal protein) in the first place. Most natural whole foods are loaded with proteins which means they are loaded with amino acids which means they are loaded with phosphorus. Sunflower seed kernels are simply the densest and since they solve four other nutrient requirements as well there is simply no reason why anyone shouldn't be eating them daily.

IODINE

In the developed countries, iodine deficiency is far higher than it should be and it is completely unnecessary. Every store that sells groceries is stocked with IODIZED SALT. 1 teaspoon a day added to anything that you cook is loaded with the IODIDE ion. It is not the best most usable form, but supplements are simply potassium iodide: the POOR FORM as well. But even though this form is not the best, since the 1920's when the government stepped in and demanded that salt brands add iodine to their products, goiter, a terrible malady that involved a MASSIVE and grotesque swelling of the thyroid and throat was virtually ELIMINATED. So we know that the IODIZED SALT does work and our bodies do manage to get enough iodine from the iodide form. The problem was that salt started to show up in everything we ate on a daily basis and often to the extreme excess (canned boiled peanuts are a perfect example of this nonsense) and thus began the medical industry's crusade to banish salt and we listened to them and now we are in trouble because very few people eat enough iodine rich foods in the U.S. and many other developed countries with the notable exception of the Japanese whose traditional diet is possibly the very healthiest on Earth.

And just because the thyroid MAKES the iodine (and selenium) based hormones, don't think that it stops there. Those hormones are then released into the bloodstream and are meant to reach EVERY CELL IN YOUR BODY to promote proper metabolism. So shorting the thyroid of iodine and selenium shorts the entire body and all cells of the critical hormones they need as well.

Rather than PAY for Potassium iodide (the form in virtually ALL supplements) just add ½ a teaspoon of IODIZED SALT to your morning oatmeal and another ½ a teaspoon somewhere else in dinner and be done with it.

MAGNESIUM

This is another nutrient found in most plant foods, but usually not in a high enough concentration to be practical. 2.5 cups of spinach per day is excessive and the ONLY SUPERFOOD loaded with it is DARK CHOCOLATE (true pure 100% CACAO mass.) Some of the "gourmet" dark chocolate bars are turning up with very high percentages of true chocolate in them, but I still prefer the good old 100% pure cacao mass found in GOOD baker's chocolate bars in the baking section of your grocery store. READ THE LABEL and if it contains more than ONE ingredient which should just read "Cacao," then it is the PROCESSED FAKE GARBAGE and DO NOT BUY THAT JUNK.

Normally I would never advocate it (just because most people think I am full of you-know-what when I do,) but I have yet to find a better source of magnesium and I do not have the patience to try to piece together a daily diet that involves ten different items each bringing 10% of a nutrient's requirement. And even if magnesium were the only benefit of this food, it would still be worth it, but it also satisfies our 100% RDA of IRON as well. Both of these are needed in relatively large amounts and 5 oz. of dark chocolate solves TWO critical requirements in one sitting. I know it sounds CRAZY but it is IMPORTANT and it is NOT candy – candy bars are so loaded up with processed JUNK that they are WORTHLESS and HARMFUL.

Dark chocolate is incredibly bitter, sweeten it with HONEY which is an amazing and powerful curative/preventative and EXCELLENT for your health too! Who would imagine that honey dipped chocolate is a HEALTH FOOD and that dark chocolate is one of the TOP SUPERFOODS on planet Earth!

WEIRD SOURCES

Some people talk about drinking a tall glass of water with a pinch of Epsom salt (Magnesium sulfate) in it or even taking a swig of Milk of Magnesia (Magnesium hydroxide) in order to get a bunch of magnesium into their system. Personally, I think both taste rather nasty and they won't solve your iron requirements either. Both are inorganic mineral forms of magnesium which makes taking magnesium in this form DUBIOUS AT BEST.

For those allergic to chocolate a little over ½ cup of pumpkin seeds contain 100% RDA of magnesium or you can take magnesium citrate which is an organic form and likely MUCH BETTER as far as availability and won't mess with your digestive system either. Milk of Magnesia neutralizes stomach acid while forming magnesium chloride, an inorganic mineral salt. And it drastically reduces your stomach's capacity to properly break down foods and KILL harmful bacteria in those foods. Epsom salt is a powerful LAXATIVE. (If you go chugging down a tall glass of that stuff and you better stay home and close to the toilet!)

ZINC

Zinc is another mineral found in most whole natural foods but in amounts that fall way short of what we need on a daily basis. I have just begun to incorporate roasted pumpkin seeds (2 cups daily) into my daily eating regimen because zinc is a critical mineral involved in countless cellular biochemical processes and has been linked to proper immune function.

Another reason that I have included it into my daily eating regimen is because virtually ALL supplements contain inorganic mineral forms that appear to have low availability. Zinc oxide is a common OTC anti-fungal powder to help fight athlete's foot, but I am not enthralled about the idea of EATING IT.

Two cups of pumpkin seeds is a lot, which is why it took me a long time to include it in my diet, and if it were not so IMPORTANT especially for proper immune function which has been linked to CANCER PREVENTION, then I wouldn't bother. Maybe there is an organic highly available product out there on the market somewhere, but I have not been able to track it down and since it is too important to ignore, I will just spend my lunch time chomping on pumpkin seeds.

OTC SUPPLEMENTS

Getting kids hooked on things like TWO CUPS of roasted pumpkin seeds per day could be difficult and in a bind a supplement might be necessary but since we do not know the availability of these inorganic forms it is nigh impossible to determine how much of it you should take for OPTIMAL THRIVE-LEVEL health. Still, something is always infinitely more than nothing at all.

SELENIUM

If you don't want to eat ½ cup of sunflower seeds each day like me, then you are in BIG TROUBLE because you are going to be forced to find natural whole food sources of your 100% RDA for vitamins B1, B5, and E as well as phosphorus and selenium. Good luck with that because all other sources are not nearly as dense as sunflower seed kernels and you will be forced to piece together dozens of different foods throughout the day to try to cover all of that. Think of them as a small handful of chewable vitamins that satisfy FIVE different CRITICAL nutrient requirements quickly and easily and in PURE biologically active and available forms too.

For those who are allergic to nuts including Brazil nuts I truly feel for you, the nuts are LOADED with excellent nutrients, the minerals in particular, and are the very best source of vitamin E which is very hard to find in reasonable quantities in any other whole natural food sources. 5 oz. of sardines will deliver 100% RDA selenium and vitamin B12 and they are a SUPERFOOD for this reason. I am not crazy about them and try to bury them in as much spicy mustard as I can, but I do eat them regularly.

One cup of pinto beans holds about 77% of your daily requirement of selenium as well. So 1.3 cups will cover it, but you MUST cook real pinto beans yourself (not canned) because we do not know how they did it and how much of the nutrients were lost in the broth while cooking them. (I will have some upcoming volumes on Healthy Cooking and Eating Right so stay tuned!)

Finally about 5 ounces of halibut will also satisfy your daily requirement of selenium, but there is some concern about eating too much of this particular species so once in a while is OK, which will fall way short of taking care of your DAILY REQUIREMENT since you should not eat it every day.

OTC SOURCES

Again, most OTC supplements that I have found are inorganic mineral forms which in a bind is better than nothing but I would greatly prefer for myself and HIGHLY RECOMMEND that you try to get your selenium from one of the many different natural forms that I have covered here. REMEMBER: selenium is for the thyroid which controls EVERY OTHER SYSTEM AND CELL IN YOUR BODY so YOU MUST get it somehow.

COPPER

Copper is an oddball and potentially DANGEROUS mineral. We do need it in small amounts but in any kind of excess it can become TOXIC. As a gardener I have read the labels of the copper sulfate treatments for plant fungus diseases and they all say that one must wear a full length rain coat with hood and a mask while spraying with the stuff to keep it from coming in contact with the skin and eyes to prevent copper metal POISONING. And virtually all OTC supplements including the big name A to Z multivitamins offer copper in a USELESS and POTENTIALLY TOXIC inorganic mineral form and I STRONGLY URGE YOU TO STAY AWAY FROM THAT JUNK.

I normally do not worry too much about copper since we only need it in trace amounts, but since we do need it; a handful of pistachios will fulfill your RDA needs in a VERY SAFE biologically active and available form. Sunflower seeds are loaded with it and the 1 cup a day regimen is practically a MEGADOSE of copper but again it is in a biological natural form which is FAR SAFER than those mineral forms so for now I am not concerned about it. In biological forms all of these substances are much more easily handled by our digestive system and eliminated easily too if they are in excess.

MANGANESE

This is yet another metal that we need in small quantities and that can be toxic in extreme excess. And again, when we get it in natural biological forms it is always FAR SAFER than in inorganic mineral forms. I do NOT RECOMMEND ANY OTC supplements of manganese for the same reason that I do NOT RECOMMEND any OTC copper supplements: THESE TWO METALS ARE POTENTIALLY VERY TOXIC and can land you in the hospital if you overdose on inorganic forms. And by the way, metal poisoning is VERY DIFFICULT TO FIX too. So the hospital will try their best but there is no real way to quickly and easily get the excesses out of your body either.

Having said that, natural and biological forms are FAR SAFER because the body can easily handle the substances and easily get rid of excesses as well. I have never heard of anyone ever getting manganese poisoning from eating too many clams or too much wheat germ and since only 1 oz. of wheat germ gives you a MIGHTY BLAST of manganese (250% RDA) then that is the way to go. I put far more than that in my morning oatmeal three to four times a week because wheat germ is a SUPERFOOD loaded with many goodies and I know it is taking care of my manganese requirements with the greatest of ease as well.

CHROMIUM

Chromium is a BIG DEAL. You MUST get it in sufficient quantities on a daily basis in order to avoid chronic deficiency which can lead you straight into SERIOUS TROUBLE called DIABETES.

Diabetes is EPIDEMIC in our country and it is very likely the most PREVALENT and most PREVENTABLE disease today. I always had hypoglycemia and tendency toward diabetes since I was a child (because everyone in my family has it.) And I am very sure that we all get it because there are simply far too many TRASH CALORIES in our normal daily eating regimen in the form of processed and packaged foods like bread, cakes, cookies, etc. AND because we are ALL suffering from CHRONIC CHROMIUM DEFICIENCY which is the root cause of the trouble.

And it is EASY to take care of our daily requirements of this CRITICAL mineral. One cup of broccoli (which I love and I know there are plenty of people who hate it) garnished with a little butter and 1 teaspoon of minced garlic (although I make it a tablespoon) and you just got all the chromium you need for the day.

Hate broccoli or don't want it daily? Three cups of 100% natural Concord grape juice per day will also solve the problem. I personally do not like the flavor of pure grape juice so I cut it half and half with ALOE VERA juice which by the way, alone tastes like DISHWASHING SOAP! But together they make each other much more mild and since BOTH have HUGE HEALTH benefits I just make sure that I drink enough to get my daily chromium requirement; three 8 oz. cups per day. That is a lot, but I used to sit down to watch football on Sunday and would knock out one 2 liter bottle of TRASH soda pop and go deep into the second one as well before the day was over. Instead, I sip on my SUPER-JUICE throughout the day and drink myself towards great health rather than toward disease and death.

OTC SUPPLEMENTS

I am obviously leery of inorganic forms and what I have found are forms like "chromium picolinate" which is an organic molecule. The medical industry however, is currently debating whether this is a usable or effective form which means they are manufacturing this nonsense and not all of the experts are convinced that even this organic molecular form is good enough. Trust me and eat your broccoli and drink your grape juice. It will keep you from ending up sick and taking very strong medications forever – once you get that DIABETES, it is very hard to CURE.

MOLYBDENUM

This metal became widely known along with vanadium in WWII as the ingredient in the supersteel used in the armor of the infamous Panzer division tanks of the German war machine. It would be decades later before we realized that both of these relatively rare metals are also essential nutrients in the human body. In fact we still do not fully understand the role vanadium plays (if any, it might just be a pervasive environmental contaminant!) and we are only beginning to understand the role of molybdenum. But ALL plants need it in trace amounts to facilitate the usage of sulfur and we need it for that reason too.

If we can't manipulate our sulfur then we can't make several amino acids that are critical components of ALL proteins and even DNA. That means that people who are suffering from chronic molybdenum deficiency will experience premature aging, systemic deterioration of all organs and systems throughout the body and are very likely much more prone to cancer. If that doesn't get your attention then nothing will. Suffice it to say, you better get some molybdenum in your diet.

I already eat oatmeal regularly and the only source I could find so far talks about the amounts in terms of calories rather than weight or volume of the food and they are also talking about "oats" and not "instant oatmeal." So my data is still rather sketchy but as an experienced gardener I know that the fast growing plants like grains are highly susceptible to molybdenum deficiency syndrome which causes mottled yellowing and upward cupping of the edges of the leaves. Since oats and "old-fashioned" oatmeal are grains that often suffer from molybdenum deficiency and require molybdenum fertilizer, I assume that all grains especially whole and unprocessed grains would have a lot of molybdenum in them.

OTC SUPPLEMENTS

There is not very much information regarding the efficacy of the molybdenum forms currently offered which are mostly inorganic forms like "sodium molybdate." Like all other metals offered in these inorganic forms I am very dubious of their effectiveness and safety and DO NOT RECOMMEND THEM. Just eat your oats and you should be fine. Green peas and lentils are also loaded with molybdenum in more than sufficient quantities to satisfy our daily requirements as well, so there are several reasonable and effective choices for everyone.

POTASSIUM

This is high on the list of minerals that most people are getting in SHORT SUPPLY on a daily basis. And potassium is nothing to fool around with either; chronic deficiency can lead to acute deficiency which causes muscle twitching, long hard bouts of hiccups and finally heart palpitations and DEATH. I believe that chronic potassium deficiency is a major contributing factor to all heart disease related DEATHS in the United States today.

And the multivitamins can't help you either because we need a HUGE AMOUNT of it on a daily basis to maintain OPTIMAL THRIVE-LEVEL health. Those 3200mg are about one heaping teaspoon of potassium chloride which means that your multivitamin pill is simply not LARGE enough to hold all of the potassium that we need and would have to be HORSE PILL sized to do it!

So I am really not exaggerating when I say that we need a LOT of potassium and if you exercise regularly which I HIGHLY ENCOURAGE EVERYONE to do, then you need EVEN MORE.

If you eat a healthy diet of whole natural foods then you are getting some potassium in all of those healthy plant foods from the oatmeal and grapefruit for breakfast to the all day snacking on trail mix of raisins, sunflower seeds and pumpkin seeds to the tossed green salad for lunch to the side of chick peas and broccoli for dinner, but it is STILL NOT ENOUGH!

That is why I URGE EVERYONE to drink at least 24 oz. of LOW SODIUM V-8 daily. That is the one item that is PACKED with potassium, enough that we can be sure we are getting 70% of what we need in a relatively small amount (I really should buy stock in that company!) Add 2 bananas and you're done.

OTC SUPPLEMENTS

While inorganic forms are probably OK, the problem is that we need so much potassium that you will find yourself swallowing pills all day long to get enough of it. I just prefer the V-8. I guess it's up to you.

SULFUR

Sulfur is found in virtually ALL natural whole foods and I normally do not worry about it very much and the FDA hasn't bothered to set a standard RDA because they feel that a well balanced and complete diet of whole foods will provide everyone with an ample supply and I tend to agree.

If you feel like you might be deficient, as long as you switch to a natural whole foods diet like everything I am recommending in these books, then you should be fine, but a couple of eggs for breakfast now and then (I eat them once a week – it is my special Sunday brunch) then you should be fine.

SODIUM and CHLORINE
I will cover these two together since they too are vital electrolytes
that our bodies need and they both come together in a very
convenient package known as salt. One teaspoon of IODIZED
SALT a day mixed into your food anywhere along the line will
ensure that you get a complete healthy dose of SODIUM,
CHLORINE AND IODINE. Just don't overdo it and remember that
if you are boiling a vegetable like broccoli in salted water that most
of the salt will stay in the liquid, so you will have to drink it. I do,
and I make sure I get all of the nutrients from the vegetable that
leeched out in the boiling process and I make sure to get the rest
of my daily REQUIREMENTS of SODIUM, CHLORINE AND
IODINE too.
COBALT
All green plants need cobalt in trace quantities but they do not
make vitamin B12 with it. That's why you must get your vitamin
B12 from an ANIMAL SOURCE. It is very likely that the herbivores
use those trace quantities found in all plants to manufacture their
vitamin B12 and even we can do that too. As far as the scientific
community now knows, that is the extent of our needs for cobalt
and as long as you are getting a good supply of B12 from natural
foods you should be fine. Also if you are eating a healthy natural
whole foods diet that includes a lot of plants like I am suggesting in
these books then you are very likely getting your fill of organic
cobalt that is not already in vitamin B12 form.

    END OF CHAPTER QUIZ
1. Name two SUPERFOODS that each bring 100% of our RDA
requirements of at least TWO different minerals that are otherwise
difficult to get enough of:
    A. Spirulina and kelp
    B. Brazil nuts and yogurt
    C. Pistachios and almonds
    D. Sunflower seeds and dark chocolate
    Answer: D. ½ cup of Sunflower seeds knocks out phosphorus
    and selenium and 5 oz. dark chocolate takes care of iron and
    magnesium (two of the hardest ones to cover.) The rest are all
    excellent sources of minerals and vitamins too.
2. The easiest way to get calcium and one of the SUPERFOODS
that provides 100% RDA of it is:
    A. Whole milk
    B. Yogurt
    C. Cheese
    D. Either B or C
    Answer: D. Two cups of yogurt or 5 oz. of cheese each day
    will supply you 100% of the RDA of calcium and yogurt is one
    of the most concentrated sources of calcium of any food and

as a SUPERFOOD also provides many other nutrients and health benefits.

3. A chronic deficiency in this mineral could lead to diabetes:
A. Zinc
B. Iron
C. Selenium
D. Chromium
Answer: D. Chromium plays a vital role in energy metabolism and insulin pathways

4. Chronic deficiency in the following could lead to a severely compromised immune system which could lead to cancer:
A. Zinc
B. Iron
C. Selenium
D. Chromium
Answer: A. Zinc has been recently linked to proper immune function and chronic deficiency could severely weaken the immune system opening the door to cancer amongst a host of other ailments and diseases.

4. Most of the world's population suffers from chronic deficiency in this mineral which can lead to chronic anemia and a host of health issues.
A. Zinc
B. Iron
C. Selenium
D. Chromium
Answer: B. Most people on the planet simply do not eat enough of the right kinds of foods on a daily basis to get enough iron. Just 3 oz. of Spirulina or 5 oz. of pure 100% dark chocolate can provide 100% RDA of iron.

5. Which of the following has no convenient superfood loaded with it forcing us to eat a lot of the best choices out there?
A. Zinc
B. Iron
C. Selenium
D. Chromium
Answer A. Zinc is too important to ignore and the food with the highest concentration, pumpkin seeds, still takes TWO CUPS to cover our daily 100% RDA of it.

7. These two minerals are simply too toxic to risk taking in inorganic supplement forms:
A. Sodium and Chlorine
B. Copper and Manganese
C. Iodine and Selenium
D. Calcium and Iron
Answer: B. Copper and Manganese excess especially in inorganic forms could lead to dangerous metal poisoning.

It is important to realize that we have no idea of ALL of the molecules present in one simple apple. And you can bet we may NEVER know either.

Think about this. It took serious technological advancements in optics to build microscopes capable of even seeing bacteria for the first time and even then they were nothing but tiny dots on a background of relatively huge eukaryotic cells (everything that isn't a bacteria is a eukaryote, so human blood cells are eukaryotic, for example.)

And these barely perceptible organisms have cilia; hairs that they SPIN with tiny organic electrical motors in order to swim. Machinery that is difficult to see in our most powerful modern scanning electron microscopes that have resolutions up to a hundred times better. The simplest little bacterium is made up of literally thousands of different kinds of molecules possibly MILLIONS. And each of those different kinds of molecules excluding water, is present in staggering numbers, possibly BILLIONS each. And that all has to be assembled exactly right in order to get a WORKING, FUNCTIONING, LIVING CELL.

The COMPLEXITY of the simplest organisms on Earth is MIND-BOGGLING. If an atom were the size of a ping-pong ball these tiny organisms would be the size of a state county. And they are the SIMPLE ones. Then there are huge organisms like the paramecium and the amoeba, far more sophisticated and complicated and to scale they would be the size of the United States. Then there are humans. Every cell in our bodies is as sophisticated as an amoeba and we are made out of thousands of different KINDS of cells and countless TRILLIONS of them. On the same scale a human body would likely be the size of a dwarf galaxy!

And down at the cellular level it all comes down to chemistry and the interactions of molecules; uncountable billions of them… in EACH CELL. So, we do know a lot more than we did prior to the renaissance when diseases were thought to be either the wrath of God or the work of the devil (and they still could be, we just know the shape of the bullets they are using on us now!) But we are a LONG way from knowing the New York telephone directory sized list of all molecules in the human body and what they do and how they ALL interact with ALL of the others and how all of those interactions result in LIFE itself.

The point? We may NEVER know ALL of the nutrients required by the human body. And we certainly have only just begun to explore the vast pharmacopoeia of "active" ingredients found in plants and animals worldwide: molecules that have preventative and curative powers beyond our wildest dreams.

Our own digestive systems and cellular processes are truly amazing in that we can manufacture MOST of the molecules we need for ourselves by breaking down what we eat into simpler building blocks that get sent throughout the body in the blood and get absorbed by the cells which then put them back together into the molecules they need.

But there are many molecules that our bodies CANNOT manufacture for themselves like VITAMIN C that if we don't get it in our diet we will get sick and die. We know about Vitamin C because we need a lot of it and it is not found in all foods, so in the old days people did get sick and die from scurvy until we discovered the connection between that disease and citrus fruits and that's why English sailors made sure to carry a supply of limes on their sailing ships and thus came to be called "Limeys." Later, we would discover why citrus fruits kept them from getting scurvy: the vitamin C within them.

But back then we had no idea that something called Omega-3 fatty acid even existed or that we can't make it in our bodies and yet we do NEED IT. And it is not something like selenium that is needed in micrograms (MILLIONTHS of a gram) either. Humans need at least 1000 milligrams (ONE whole gram) of it daily and possibly MORE than that to achieve OPTIMAL THRIVE-LEVEL health.

And we certainly can't make salicylic acid (aspirin) but it does work to sooth pain. And the list of modern wonder drugs discovered in plants is vast; most of our modern medicines were originally discovered in plants used by local indigenous communities around the world for centuries before our science decided to investigate them.

It makes me wonder, in sixty years will some newly discovered essential nutrient be all the rage and all of the food manufacturers and pill makers will be putting that molecule's name in bold on their products just like "Omega-3" is now? You can bet on it.

In the meantime, what can we do to ensure that we are getting ALL of the essential nutrients our bodies need including those we haven't even discovered yet? The answer is very simple: stop trying to live on a George Jetson diet of manufactured GARBAGE and PILLS and start eating natural whole foods. Those foods are what our species was eating before we even became our species and if they were good enough to transform us from simians into scientists, then they are still good enough to transform us from scientists into whatever will come next.

And a varied diet of ONLY natural whole foods will contain everything the human body needs. If that were not the case then we would never have survived at all; much less have been able to EVOLVE into a higher form of life. That process REQUIRES A LOT MORE ENERGY than just languishing along and barely surviving; it requires OPTIMAL and THRIVE-LEVEL health. And the reason the world is NOT at that level now is not because the foods aren't good enough: it is because the manmade GARBAGE most people are eating IS NOT GOOD ENOUGH and is in fact USELESS if not outright POISONOUS.

The only difference between a bag of potato chips and a rattlesnake bite is the TIME IT TAKES TO KILL YOU. But they BOTH DO.

If you eat nothing but natural whole foods then the likelihood that you are getting ALL of the essential (those things we cannot manufacture in our bodies) nutrients is nearly 100% even for those nutrients we have yet to discover because where else could they be? And if you WASTE THE TIME, MONEY and EFFORT to load up on packaged processed foods then you will NOT be getting enough of these essential nutrients and you will suffer chronic deficiencies of just about all of them. I am often amazed that I even survived based on what I ate from the age of 15 to 25 years old. But I was in terrible shape and that was when I started to change and that is a very good thing because I know I would not be alive today if I hadn't. Iron and Chromium deficiencies alone would have buried me long ago.

There are unknown constituents in virtually ALL natural whole foods and as a species we were raised on these foods, they didn't just keep us alive, they were good enough for us to THRIVE and EVOLVE and the whole modern attitude that the George Jetson lifestyle is superior because we think we are so smart that we can make food that is better than nature is both ARROGANT and ABSURD. Oh, we are pretty clever apes, but we have only been doing science for about 450 years, but we have been eating nature's bounty and doing very well on it for MILLIONS of years. Maybe someday the scientists will be able to make a George Jetson diet for us that really works, but that is a LONG WAY OFF.

Now, lets take a look at the rest of the essential nutrients that we must get in our diet.

Name	TYPE	RDA
Isoleucine	Amino acid	≈110g*
Histidine	Amino acid	≈110g*
Leucine	Amino acid	≈110g*
Lysine	Amino acid	≈110g*
Methionine	Amino acid	≈110g*
Phenylalanine	Amino acid	≈110g*
Tryptophan	Amino acid	≈110g*
Threonine	Amino acid	≈110g*
Valine	Amino acid	≈110g*
alpha-linolenic acid (ALA)	Omega-3	>1000mg*
docosahexaenoic acid (DHA)	Omega-3	>1000mg*
eicosapentaenoic acid (EPA)	Omega-3	>1000mg*

* Experts argue that we need a MINIMUM of 500mg of Omega-3 daily, but of which ones? The current recommendation is that we should get about 110 grams of protein daily and it should contain all NINE of the ESSENTIAL AMINO acids. That's FOUR OUNCES MINIMUM. I would like to see George Jetson swallow THAT pill.
We still do not know what the RDA should be for any of these essential nutrients. The Omega-3's are complicated because there are at least three different ones that we have identified so far and we know that we can convert ALA into DHA and EPA, but we do not know how efficient the body is at this process and we don't know how much of those we need for OPTIMUM THRIVE-LEVEL health. But first, let's take a look at all of those amino acids.

First, the NINE ESSENTIAL AMINO ACIDS are all found in protein rich foods and animal meat is NUMBER ONE for providing them. But there is no need to despair; most can also be found in protein rich plant foods as well. Animal sources do contain ALL nine, but many plants contain very little methionine and lysine which is why vegetarians need to make sure they are getting enough of those two amino acids in particular.

ISOLEUCINE

This amino acid is critical to the formation of hemoglobin in the blood and also helps muscle growth in children in particular. KIDS NEED A LOT OF PROTEIN, adults need it too because most of our organ systems are constantly in the process of regeneration and renewal and therefore constantly engaged in cell division and growth. Amino acid (protein) deficient diets low in isoleucine lead to slow development and poor overall health as well as progressive degeneration of all bodily systems and premature aging notably in the skin and hair, but also reduced brain function and weakened and inflamed joints.[14]

HISTIDINE

Foods high in histidine (again found in most protein rich foods) assist in detoxification of the body and proper brain function.[14]

LEUCINE

Leucine has been shown to help regulate insulin and therefore normalize blood sugar levels. People who are eating a low protein diet or suffer from chronic leucine deficiency are at risk and this can play a contributing role in the development of diabetes or hypoglycemia. If you haven't noticed yet, BLOOD SUGAR and its proper function is one of the MOST COMPLEX systems in the human body and there is a VAST number of essential nutrients and other biochemical processes and organ systems at work to keep it running properly. This is indeed one system in our body that we LIVE or DIE on and it has a LOT of moving parts. A healthy balanced natural whole foods diet is the very best way to make sure that none of those gears in that massive and complicated system gets fouled up.[14]

LYSINE

Lysine has been shown to play a critical role in the body's proper usage of CALCIUM and supports proper bone health. All of the CONCRETE tablets on Earth WILL NOT prevent osteoporosis without LYSINE (proper all natural whole foods diet rich in animal protein) although they should be able to give you a baseball sized kidney stone quickly enough.[14]

METHIONINE

This is one of the amino acids that contains sulfur. You would expect to find it in the sulfurous foods like eggs and broccoli and you would be quite right. Methionine is critical to the construction and maintenance of cartilage in the body and why people on low protein diets get joint problems QUICKLY.[14]

PHENYLALANINE

Try to say THAT three times fast. Phenylalanine (I remember it as "fennil-ala-neen") is critical to thyroid health and helps the gland produce its hormones, the ones built on those two weird minerals already discussed: iodine and selenium. Low protein diets consisting of mostly GARBAGE calories in packaged and processed foods can also reduce thyroid function and land you in a world of trouble with lower metabolism and obesity. Overweight people who also have a problem staying warm (often complain about the "freezing" temperature in an air-conditioned office) ARE SUFFERING FROM SEVERELY REDUCED METABOLIC RATE caused by DEPRESSED THYROID FUNCTION. You can piece everything together from these books but I will include an upcoming volume on this global epidemic problem and how you can EASILY FIX IT.[14]

TRYPTOPHAN

Often thought of as the reason we get drowsy after eating a ton of turkey on Thanksgiving, that drowsiness is actually caused by the very high levels of LACTIC ACID in turkey meat. LACTIC ACID is what your body produces as a by-product of lengthy exercise and what makes your muscles ache and makes you feel exhausted. Tryptophan is an essential amino acid incorporated into every protein in every cell of your body and virtually all high protein foods have just as much as turkey, so let's get that TRUTH taken care of once and for all shall we: LACTIC ACID; NOT TRYPTOPHAN. (Obviously I am tired of arguing about this with everyone. I don't know where that DISINFORMATION started, but it is time to put a stop to it already.) Tryptophan is involved in proper neuro-transmitter and brain function. Ironically it makes you MORE ALERT and improves concentration, mood, etc. It has the opposite effect of lactic acid. And chicken has MORE tryptophan than turkey so it is NOT the Tryptophan. OK, I'm done with my rant.[14]

THREONINE

This amino acid is also linked to proper central nervous system function as well as heart, liver and immune health. A chronic low protein diet could land you in BIG TROUBLE if you are putting all of those systems at risk.[14]

VALINE

Body-builders know what valine is for: proper muscle growth, strength and endurance. Even though we do not necessarily want to look like those guys (and gals!) we still need it for proper muscle formation and maintenance.[14]

TOP FOODS RICH IN THE NINE ESSENTIAL AMINO ACIDS

By the way there are plenty more amino acids than this, but our bodies can build them mainly by modifying these, so we cannot scrimp on these ESSENTIAL (means: we don't make them or we can't make enough of them to satisfy our bodily requirements of them on a daily basis) NUTRIENTS.

EGGS – Body builders know all about the power of eggs. They are one of the densest sources of animal protein foods on Earth and are LOADED with all NINE ESSENTIAL AMINO acids along with the B vitamins and some minerals as well. One large egg holds 6g of protein. This seems a little low to me, but that's what the experts say they have. Three for breakfast have set you up with about 1/6 of your daily protein requirement in a VERY RICH whole natural food source.[14]

CHEESE – Preferably unprocessed, all-natural cheese. Parmesan cheese happens to be loaded with protein and all nine essential amino acids. Low fat cheddar tips the scales with 28g of protein per ounce (it is almost PURE PROTEIN (an ounce is about 28.35 grams.) But all cheeses are high in protein ranging from about 22 to 28 grams of protein per ounce. 5 ounces of just about any solid natural cheese will cover your minimum daily requirement for high quality protein containing all nine essential amino acids. Cheese is the NUMBER ONE PROTEIN SUPERFOOD.[14]

YOGURT – This is a SUPERFOOD loaded with vitamins and minerals and Complete Protein (all nine essential amino acids.) One cup of low fat yogurt holds about 14 grams. Two cups (which fulfill your CALCIUM daily requirement in the healthiest and highest density form) knock out about ¼ of your RDA of complete protein.[14]

POULTRY – Animal meat is also a SUPERFOOD and MOSTLY complete protein as well. Chicken and turkey are no less than 70% complete protein, so 4 to 6 ounces will cover your RDA of the nine essential amino acids.[14]

LAMB – Very dense and complete animal protein packed with many other hard to get vitamins and minerals. Lamb is a true SUPERFOOD and 4 to 6 ounces will definitely cover your RDA of complete protein.[14]

BEEF – Almost as dense as Lamb, just 4 to 6 ounces will cover your RDA of complete protein.[14]

FISH – This is another animal flesh PACKED with complete protein. Just 4 to 6 ounces of just about any species will fulfill your daily requirements for complete protein AND many other vitamins minerals and the OMEGA-3 fatty acids as well. This is precisely why I consider all FISH in general to be SUPERFOODS.[14]

FOR VEGETARIANS

MOST plant protein falls short in methionine and lysine. The sulfurous plants like broccoli and cauliflower have the methionine as does garlic, but you certainly don't want to sit down to a meal of garlic and that still leaves lysine as a real issue. Personally speaking and I know I won't convince any vegan to do it, but a 5 oz. block of low fat cheddar will easily solve the Complete Protein and Calcium daily requirement and added bonus; they don't kill the cows to make it either.[14]

LENTILS – 1 cup provides about 18g of protein.

GREEN PEAS – 1 cup provides about 16.5g protein.

CHICK PEAS – 1 cup provides about 15g protein.

PEANUT BUTTER – 1oz provides about 7g of protein. Peanut butter is a very dense source of protein and I highly recommend it although it also brings a lot of calories, but they are in the form of polyunsaturated fats (the good kind.)

PEANUTS – roughly the same as peanut butter, about 7g per ounce. Obviously the legumes are all loaded with protein.

SUNFLOWER SEEDS – 5.5g per ounce. One cup of kernels (about 6 to 7 ounces) brings about 33 to 39 grams of protein or roughly 1/3 of your daily protein requirements. This SUPERFOOD will also bring you 100% RDA of Vitamins B1, B5 and E and Phosphorus and Selenium.

PUMPKIN SEEDS – 8.5g per ounce. Pumpkin seeds are loaded with protein. TWO CUPS which solve the ZINC requirement and weigh about 10 to 14 ounces and bring 100% RDA of protein for the day as well, but remember that these plant sources are NOT COMPLETE PROTEIN (which contains sufficient amounts of ALL NINE essential amino acids.)

THE OMEGA-3 FATTY ACIDS

We need these and currently experts are divided as to how much constitutes a healthy daily amount. This is further aggravated by the fact that infants, children, adolescents, men, women, and pregnant/nursing mothers may all need significantly different quantities for ideal health. Currently the studies are on-going and we will eventually know the facts, but in the meantime EVERYONE needs all three (that we have identified so far) and we need a LOT of it in our daily eating regimen.

While I have no major quarrel with the plethora of fish oil and krill oil products on the market today, I am still a major proponent of getting our nutrients in their NATURAL states, in natural whole foods, because those foods contain other constituents that often act as digestive buffers and even catalysts that assist in the absorption of those nutrients. And whole fish are no exception. I have found at least one article that talks about the presence of another compound in the fish that does assist in the absorption of the Omega-3 fatty acids. So eating the foods in the natural forms IS FAR BETTER FOR YOU than gulping down a large pill once or twice a day.

Of further and CRITICAL importance is the fact that the RATIO of Omega-6 fatty acid to Omega-3 fatty acids seems to have a profound effect on the benefits of the Omega-3's. To wit, a daily diet high in Omega-6's (vegetable oils are LOADED with it including my favorite, Canola oil) DIMINISHES the benefits of the Omega-3's.

As such it is imperative to LOWER our intake of these GOOD POLYUNSATURATED vegetable oils and INCREASE our intake of the OMEGA-3 FATTY ACIDS.[15]

WHAT ARE THE OMEGA-3 FATTY ACIDS GOOD FOR?
We know that they are essential nutrients, which means that the human body needs them and we cannot make them ourselves and they have to be in our diet. We know that the Omega-3's are necessary for heart health and that chronic deficiency can and will lead to heart disease and ultimately a heart attack.

While anecdotal, just consider this: my father despised fish and didn't even want it cooked in the house because of its "wretched stench." He also had four heart attacks and a stroke and the last heart attack killed him. He was otherwise a very healthy, tough old dog who ate just about everything else you can imagine in abundance like broccoli, liver (which he LOVED) and so on. I am not saying that the TOTAL LACK of Omega-3 killed him, but the evidence is mounting for that case.

Chronic deficiency of Omega-3 can have dire consequences including: inflammation as well as allergies, higher risk for heart disease, higher risk for high cholesterol, digestive disorders, joint and muscle pain as well as full-blown arthritis, poor brain development that can lead to cognitive decline and mental disorders like depression. Clearly I want no part of any of that and I suspect that chronic deficiency is the NUMBER ONE ROOT CAUSE OF HIGH CHOLESTEROL in the United States today because Americans are BEEF EATERS and not FISH EATERS like the Japanese who happen to be FAR HEALTHIER than every other society on the planet.

The benefits of getting proper amounts of Omega-3 in your diet are equally amazing and include: improves and maintains cardiovascular health by lowering blood pressure, cholesterol, plaque buildup in the arteries, and the chance of having a heart attack or stroke; helps stabilize blood sugar levels (preventing diabetes, yet another gear in the amazingly complicated blood sugar balance and utilization machinery); reduces muscle, bone and joint pain by lowering inflammation; sharpens the mind and helps with concentration and learning; improves mood and prevents depression; boosts the immune system; helps treat digestive disorders like ulcerative colitis; reduces risk for cancer and helps prevent cancer reoccurrence.[15]

GETTING YOUR DAILY OMEGA-3'S

Almost all plant sources contain ONLY ALA (Alpha-Linoleic acid) which is certainly better than nothing at all, but a VERY POOR SECOND CHOICE to getting a sizeable and OPTIMAL AND THRIVE-LEVEL amount of DHA and EPA on a daily basis and those are ONLY found in FISH (and other sea creatures.)

Growing up in South Florida you can bet we learned how to fish and most natives love their seafood ranging from fish, to shrimp, to crab, to lobster. And I would never complain if that was all I ever ate for dinner for the rest of my life. I have fish at least twice a week sometimes much more than that and I am trying to make it my daily lunch and/or dinner and so should you.[15]

OMEGA-3 FOODS:

ATLANTIC MACKEREL: ≈1,000 milligrams per ounce. This is THE Omega-3 (DHA/EPA) SUPERFOOD with the highest concentration on Earth.

COD LIVER OIL: 2.664mg per tablespoon. Cod liver oil is not exactly a food, but it does have the HIGHEST concentration of Omega-3 (DHA/EPA) of any natural substance on Earth and it is also loaded with Vitamins A and D.

WALNUTS: ≈1,300mg per ounce (ALA ONLY.)

CHIA SEEDS: 2,457mg per tablespoon. This is the highest concentration of Omega-3 albeit ALA of all plant food sources.

ALASKAN SALMON (wild-caught): ≈575mg per ounce (DHA/EPA)

FLAXSEEDS (ground): 1,597mg per tablespoon (ALA.)

ALBACORE TUNA: ≈470mg per ounce (DHA/EPA)

SARDINES: ≈360mg per ounce (DHA/EPA)

Tuna and sardines are SUPERFOODS and both are cheap so there is no reason why everybody can't add them to their eating regimen and start getting these ESSENTIAL Omega-3 fatty acids into their diet. They are simply TOO IMPORTANT TO IGNORE.

END OF CHAPTER QUIZ

1. Which amino acid is linked to neurotransmitter and brain function?

    A. Tryptophan

    B. Leucine

    C. Lysine

    D. Phenylalanine

    Answer: A. Tryptophan has been linked to proper function of neurotransmitters and helps with cognitive brain function and leads to having a sharper and more alert mind, It DOES NOT make you drowsy contrary to popular belief.

2. Which amino acid is linked to proper blood sugar regulation and can thus help mitigate or possibly even prevent diabetes?

    A. Tryptophan

B. Leucine
C. Lysine
D. Phenylalanine
Answer: B. Leucine has been linked to proper function of insulin in the human body and a healthy natural whole food diet that includes excellent sources of COMPLETE PROTEIN can help mitigate and possibly even prevent diabetes.

3. Which amino acid is linked to the proper absorption of CALCIUM and the maintenance of healthy bones?
    A. Tryptophan
    B. Leucine
    C. Lysine
    D. Phenylalanine
Answer: C. Lysine helps the body absorb calcium and manage it properly and promotes strong and healthy bones.

4. Which amino acid has been linked to the thyroid's ability to produce its all-important hormones?
    A. Tryptophan
    B. Leucine
    C. Lysine
    D. Phenylalanine
Answer: D. Phenylalanine. A chronic lack of COMPLETE protein in the diet can still lead to serious thyroid gland issues even if the person is getting enough iodine and selenium.

5. Which Omega-3 can be found in plant matter but it is FAR FROM IDEAL to have a diet limited only to this form?
    A. Docosahexaenoic acid (DHA)
    B. Eicosapentaenoic acid (EPA)
    C. Alpha-linoleic acid (ALA)
    D. L-ascorbic acid
Answer: C. Alpha-linolenic acid (ALA). It is critical that a person get DHA and EPA in their daily diet because we do not yet know how efficient the human body is at manufacturing these from ALA.

6. Which natural food product has the highest concentration of DHA and EPA Omega-3's of all?
    A. Atlantic mackerel
    B. Cod liver oil
    C. Chia seeds
    D. Walnuts
Answer: B. Cod liver oil. Just one tablespoon per day will give you over 2,500mg of the good Omega-3's. I DESPISED this stuff as a kid, but for those who have cardiovascular health issues and don't want to eat mackerel, this is your NUMBER ONE alternative.

THE GOOD FOODS LIST – PRIMARY FOODS

I provide this kind of a list in volumes 1 and 2, but to recap quickly:

1. **RAW EDIBLE VEGETABLES** – Anything that can be eaten raw including all of the green leafy vegetables from lettuce and cabbage and their kin, to celery to carrots, to onions and garlic are all exceptionally healthy foods loaded with nutrients.

2. **FRUITS** – The vast majority are loaded with vitamin C along with many other essential nutrients and other constituents that are currently being investigated that have a wide range of health benefits.

3. **NUTS** – These are loaded with Vitamin E and many different minerals depending on the type of nut. Although they are high in fat, it is the good kind, polyunsaturated fat, but they still pack a lot of calories and are not the best friend to the person trying to lose weight.

4. **SEEDS** – Sunflower seeds are the KING of the SEED foods. They are a SUPERFOOD and highly recommended. Pumpkin seeds and pine nuts are also loaded with essential nutrients and are highly recommended as well.

5) **YOGURT** – This is a very healthy alternative to ice cream. I buy it plain and add my own fruits, nuts and seeds to it or sometimes I buy it with the fruits already added.

6) **FISH** – Sardines, salmon, and tuna are all loaded with essential nutrients, but ALL fish are very healthy foods and the number one source of animal protein which our bodies need.

7) **POULTRY** – Chicken and turkey meat (skinned to remove most of the saturated fats) are the second healthiest animal protein you can eat and should be part of a regular daily eating regimen.

8) **FRUIT AND VEGETABLE JUICES** – Replace soda pop and other junk food drinks with these healthy and refreshing alternatives. ALL vegetable juices MUST be the "Low Sodium" versions. These use potassium salts to make them salty rather than sodium salts. Our bodies NEED HUGE amounts of potassium to ensure proper function of the nerve endings especially for muscle activation. Chronic low potassium is likely a contributing factor of heart failure which is the number one cause of death in the United States today. Low Sodium vegetable juices usually contain plenty of potassium and drinking two servings per day could SAVE YOUR HEART AND YOUR LIFE.

THE BAD FOODS LIST

1) **PROCESSED FOODS** – Anything in a box or a plastic bag made from processed grain flour and/or laced with artificial flavors, colors, preservatives and so on (See Chapter 1 of Vol.2.)

2. **SODA POP** – Most of these nuisances contain NOTHING THAT WAS EVER ALIVE. The mild carbonic acid which gives them their

fizz, is NO GOOD FOR YOU OR YOUR DIGESTIVE TRACT and most are laced with artificial colors and flavors. (They don't need preservatives because even the bacteria want no part of them!) Eliminate this GARBAGE from your diet. Drink vegetable and fruit juices instead as well as plenty of water which is the number one liquid you can drink for better health anyway.

3. **CANDY** – This crud is ALL awful. Eat fruits instead. Many are just as sweet as candy but contain FRUCTOSE which is a very healthy form of sugar that your body does need in order to function. Your brain runs on glucose; no sugar = pass out. Ask anyone who suffers from hypoglycemia or diabetes and they can tell you all about it. Fructose must be converted into glucose which slows down its absorption and arrival in the blood stream.

THE SECONDARY FOODS – SHOULD BE DRAMATICALLY REDUCED IN A HEALTHY DIET

1) **GRAINS** – Most people think I am a lunatic when I call these BAD FOODS, and they are not totally evil, but anything that has to be cooked in order to become edible is definitely on the SECONDARY FOOD list which means I do not eat them regularly as a group. Foods made from processed grains like white flour are a definite EVIL and BAD FOR YOU. I apologize to all of the bakers out there, but until they start making WHOLE GRAIN 100% WHEAT FLOUR donuts and cookies sweetened with fruit sugar or honey, I must insist that I am right here. There are a few exceptions to each rule: see the exception list below.

2) **STARCHY ROOTS** – Anything that must be cooked in order to make it edible including potatoes, yucca, malanga, boniato, etc. I know this is bad news for the Hispanics and trust me I miss them sorely too, but the TRUTH is that these foods are ALL very HIGH in calories, and while some may bring some essential nutrients, they are simply not enough to justify the TONS of CALORIES they bring. I eat them very sparingly.

3) **BEANS** – And any other vegetable foods that must be cooked in order to make them edible are all on the SECONDARY FOODS list: eat them very sparingly.

SECONDARY FOODS (SHOULD BE REDUCED) THAT ARE NOT SO EVIL AS YOU THINK

1) **EGGS** – Maligned for decades since the discovery of cholesterol and its link to heart disease, eggs are NOT going to kill you unless you eat them raw or by the dozen. I have three eggs over easy for breakfast about once a week. But my cholesterol is under control. If yours is high you should stay away until you have it under control and PLEASE DO NOT TAKE THOSE TERRIBLE DRUGS TO DO IT (See the upcoming volume on taking control of your Cholesterol without DRUGS.)

2. **DAIRY** – I realize that this is a SECONDARY FOOD and many people are developing lactose intolerance. This is due mainly to OVERINDULGENCE and its presence in far too great a quantity in

the average American diet. I use a little in my coffee and make one café con leche each day, so my daily intake is a little over 1 cup a day of whole milk. Cheeses and even butter is fine although I prefer the cheap margarines which are mostly vegetable oil anyway. By the way, I know a lot of people that have switched to 2% skim milk or even 1% and 0% (which tastes like white colored water to me.) Do you know the percentage fat content of whole milk? Most people guess 20% to 50% when I ask them this question and I have to laugh. Do you realize that Half and Half has roughly this percentage of fat? "Whole milk" is an advertising term that started when people COMPLAINED about the fact that the milk had all of the cream removed and then it was pasteurized and homogenized and to them (back then) it tasted like 0% skim milk tastes to me now. Modern "Whole milk" which has had most of the cream removed is about 3% to 5% fat. They aren't going to leave much in it because they can sell that cream in the form of cheese and butter and Half and Half at a premium.

3) **BEEF** – Often blamed for causing high cholesterol as well, beef is also not nearly as evil as people now believe. Beef is high in many essential nutrients and the only source of some animal amino acids for most people unless they also eat poultry and fish. Beef liver, which is an organ, and not the beef meat, is one of natures true SUPERFOODS and it is LOADED with vitamins and minerals and is excellent for you (even if it does make me gag.)

4) PORK – Yes, this one is a bit high in saturated fat and cholesterol so if you are having issues with your weight or with cholesterol then you should definitely avoid pork until you have that under control. If you never eat it again in life, the Jews will let you into their synagogues and you probably wouldn't miss a beat on your way to a longer and healthier life, but it certainly won't kill you if you eat it sparingly. I have some sliced pink ham in a sandwich or for breakfast about once a month, and pork chops for dinner about once a month.

NOTABLE EXCEPTIONS TO THE RULES

1) **OATMEAL** – Even though this is a grain and would normally be considered a SECONDARY FOOD (to be eaten very sparingly) OATMEAL happens to be an excellent "curative" or "preventative" food for the heart. Because it promotes heart health, I advise oatmeal as the ONLY cereal to eat for breakfast. I prefer the regular old-fashioned oats to the instant just because the instant has been "messed with" or processed in some way in order to make it instant. True natural oatmeal is the food that is good for your heart and we do not know how much of its effectiveness has been lost by tampering with it to make it instant. And it doesn't matter that much since regular old oatmeal boils up in about 8 to 12 minutes anyway. I have it at least four times a week.

2. CHICK PEAS (GARBANZOS) – A true SECONDARY FOOD by definition that must be cooked in order to be edible (raw chick

peas are harder than human teeth, you would literally chip, crack and split your teeth trying to eat them raw!) Nevertheless, cooked chick peas are loaded with nutrients and good to eat although I still hold them down to about once a week.

3) **GREEN PEAS** – Another legume that is loaded with nutrients and OK to eat on occasion.

4) **LENTILS** – These too should be SECONDARY FOODS and eaten sparingly but they have plenty of nutrients in them as well.

5) **PEANUTS** – Technically legumes and not a form of nut, they are sort of "in-betweeners" because they do have some nut-like properties including the fact that they are loaded with fat and therefore calories. But they do also have high nutrient content as well. Not the dieter's friend but a snack only when you have nothing else to eat such as a peanut butter sandwich which can get you through to dinner.

THE SUPERFOODS

I try to stick to these as much as possible for two reasons: 1) They guarantee that you will get all of the nutrient that your body needs on a daily basis, and 2) Globally, I believe that High Intensity Agriculture and Animal Husbandry have reached the point that most foods are experiencing a drastic reduction in their nutritional content. In other words, all of those oats are growing in long dead moon dust and if they do not get a continual supply of fertilizer, and irrigation they would shrivel up and die quickly. And trace essential nutrients for plants like molybdenum are extremely expensive (molybdenum compounds cost six times more than the same weight of solid silver) so I know farmers will never apply it until the plants are showing outward symptoms of molybdenum deficiency. Since all plants need trace amounts of it, then it is fair to assume that all plants grown in that DEAD moon dust soil are deficient. And because we are first and foremost vegetarians all the way back to our humble evolutionary beginnings, then it should be obvious that we need it too.

Because of this I believe that ALL nutrients, minerals in particular, are now severely diminished in all of our natural foods. Even a 50% reduction from the late 1800's to now would mean the difference between a particular food in a reasonable portion size having enough of a particular nutrient to satisfy the average person's daily requirement and now falling way short of the mark. And this is exactly why I have had to trim most lists of foods when I look up "Foods high in X" because the majority of them list reasonably sized portions and then they say they have 10% of our daily requirement of the nutrient in them. To me this is a waste of time. Should I eat a dozen eggs of a whole bushel of beans during the day? My goal is NOT to get SOME of the nutrient that I need on a daily basis (that is the definition of chronic deficiency which we are all suffering from in the first place,) rather it is to get ALL of

the nutrient my body needs on a daily basis. The SUPERFOODS
will help ensure that this goal is met with ease.

This book covers the minerals, essential amino acids and the
Omega-3 fatty acids so I am concentrating on them here, but in
the volume on vitamins, some of these superfoods show up there
as well because they contain some of those in abundance as well
(and that's why some of them are SUPERFOODS.) Therefore, I
will point out that these superfoods bring far more than just those
nutrients I am listing in this particular book in the series and are
very much well worth the effort of being included into your daily
eating regimen.

1) **CHEESE** – 5 ounces of just about any unprocessed cheese will
meet your MINIMUM RDA for COMPLETE protein containing
ample amounts of all NINE ESSENTIAL amino acids. It is also
loaded with CALCIUM and Vitamin D.

2) **YOGURT** – Two cups a day will fulfill your CALCIUM RDA and
satisfy about ¼ of your daily requirement of COMPLETE protein.
Good quality organic yogurt can also fulfill 100% of your daily
requirements of IODINE.

3) **SPIRULINA** – There is no other food source on planet Earth as
high in iron as this blue-green algae. Just 3 ounces will satisfy your
RDA for iron which is much harder to do than most people think.
Beef liver has the highest concentration of iron of all beef products
and it takes about a POUND to get all the iron you need.

4) **DARK CHOCOLATE** – Don't like the taste of spirulina? Or
maybe you don't relish the idea of eating a POUND of beef liver
daily? 5 ounces of pure 100% CACAO mass will satisfy your RDA
of iron as well as magnesium which is another mineral that is
difficult to get in sufficient quantities. Given the choice I will
blissfully eat my dark chocolate rather than gag on spirulina for the
rest of my OPTIMAL and THRIVE-LEVEL iron-rich life.

5) **SUNFLOWER SEEDS** – ½ cup of kernels a day gives you
100% RDA of Phosphorus and Selenium. It also provides you with
roughly 100% of the RDA of Vitamins B1, B5 and E and also
provides about 50% of the RDA of protein although this might be
deficient in methionine and lysine. Still sunflower seeds are the
NUMBER ONE SUPERFOOD ON EARTH.

6) **IODIZED SALT** – 1 teaspoon a day will more than fulfill your
RDA's of SODIUM which contrary to a generation of negative
HYPE, we do need, and CHLORINE and IODINE. It is not to be
confused with a health food, but if you are in doubt about your
daily intake of IODINE, just 1 teaspoon will solve that problem.

7) **PUMPKIN SEEDS** – ZINC is an important mineral that we need
in significant quantities on a daily basis for OPTIMAL and THRIVE-
LEVEL health and there is no true superfood other than LAMB and
PUMPKIN SEEDS in order to get enough daily. And it still takes
about 7 ounces of LAMB or two cups of pumpkin seeds to get it.
Still it is better than taking some cheap inorganic supplement.

PUMPKIN SEEDS are also an excellent natural source of other vitamins and minerals as well which we need in significant amounts and are far better than if taken in manufactured forms.
8) **WHEAT GERM** – What is this stuff? Plants have a very weird reproductive system. Pollen actually delivers TWO sperm cells to the ovum. One joins the ovum cell and grows into a small plant embryo in the seed, the other also joins the ovum and grows into a "germ mass" rather than a twin embryo. Within the seed, when conditions are favorable, the embryo begins to grow and it grows on the germ mass in order to swell and break out of the seed shell. The germ mass is then equivalent to an egg yolk in animal eggs. It is a SOLID MASS OF PURE NUTRIENTS for the seed embryo to grow on first to begin its life. Wheat germ basically contains almost ALL of the wheat grain's nutrients without all of the rest which is relatively devoid of most nutrients. The reason whole grain wheat bread is nutritious is because the wheat germ was kept in the creation of the whole wheat flour. I would argue that wheat germ is by far the best way to go because it is the pure chunk of nutrients within the wheat grain and should be included in your eating regimen as much as possible. I try to eat it at least four times a week. (Just add it near the end of the cooking of the oatmeal.) For those who are gluten intolerant, you will likely have to stay away from it, but that's not a problem. There are other equally nutritious foods. Get a superdose of organic and SAFE MANGANESE as well as Vitamin B7 and B9 from about 2.5 ounces. Garnish your morning oatmeal with just a little wheat germ and you are well on your way to better health for life.
9) **BROCCOLI** – I sure am glad that I LOVE broccoli. Just one cup a day will provide you with 88% of the RDA of Chromium a VITAL nutrient in blood sugar regulation that can keep you from getting diabetes. Garnish with a teaspoon of fresh minced garlic and get the other 12% you need.
10) **GRAPE JUICE** – There is some concern that grapes and grape juice are bad for your kidneys. Anyone with kidney problems should avoid grapes and their products. Otherwise monitor your kidneys and drink three 8 oz, cups of 100% pure Concord grape juice per day along with plenty of water in between. This will provide you with lots of iron and 100% RDA of Chromium. Concord grapes also contain a substance that helps slowly and safely dissolve arterial plaque so this SUPERFOOD is not just nutritious it is also a powerful, unique curative/preventative to boot!
11) **OATMEAL** – ½ cup of cooked real oatmeal (not instant) will satisfy your RDA of molybdenum. We don't need much but it is critical for our ability to utilize sulfur in our foods. No sulfur means no cellular growth or division which halts the regeneration of every tissue and organ of the body from the skin to the bones and everything in between. Oats are high in fiber (which improves digestion and many believe can treat and prevent a host of

digestive maladies including cancer) as well and that combination makes oatmeal a SUPERFOOD.

12) **LOW SODIUM VEGETABLE JUICE** – The makers of the product retain the salty flavor of their drink by using LOTS of potassium based salt and that is a VERY GOOD THING because we need a LOT of potassium on a daily basis; so much that no other food contains it in sufficient quantities to satisfy our RDA requirement of it in a quick and easy serving. 24oz. of LOW SODIUM V-8 brand will get you 70% and 2 bananas will add another 28% and finish the job.

13) **SARDINES** – Not the most popular fish on Earth I admit, but they are loaded up with vitamin B12 which is a MUST for proper BRAIN HEALTH and function which in turns leads to having and being in a PROPER MIND. I firmly believe that Vitamin B12 deficiency is the number one cause of INSANITY in our society today. If people had proper BRAIN nutrition which includes ALL of the vitamins and minerals and other essential nutrients in proper forms and amounts, I think everything from pettiness, to fear to crime would all go down. I get sardines in those flat pop top cans plain and add my own mustard or hot sauce even though they do sell them in those sauces. I just prefer my own because I know they are not laced with everything from artificial this, that, and the other or hydrogenated soy which is a DOUBLE WHAMMY EVIL. (Soy by-products are under scrutiny and suspected of being BAD for you, and partially hydrogenated ANYTHING is BAD for you.) SARDINES make the list because they are HIGH IN DHA and EPA OMEGA-3 FATTY ACIDS which are necessary for your heart and complete vascular system health.

14) **LAMB** – I wish my grocery store would carry it, but there isn't much call for it in my rather small town. It is nevertheless LOADED with nutrients and possibly the BEST animal meat as far as nutrient content goes. If you can get it and learn how to cook it, I do envy you and strongly recommend it. 7 ounces contains the RDA of Zinc, along with many of the B vitamins in ample amounts as well. Lamb is a true SUPERFOOD.

15) **SALMON** – Preferably wild-caught. The reason for this is pretty much the same as for avoiding high-intensity agricultural products: limited supply of nutrients to the end product. Fish raised on farms will almost always have a limited food supply especially in VARIETY. This in turn limits the nutritional value of the meat. Salmon are a true superfood loaded with many vitamins and DHA and EPA Omega-3 fatty acids. They are well worth including in your daily food regimen.

16) **TUNA** – Did you know that certain species of tuna are the largest bony fish on Earth? Some weigh well over a TON. They are also some of the fastest swimmers on Earth as well. Tuna is a true superfood loaded with many essential nutrients including the Omega-3 fatty acids which contribute to heart health which puts

tuna at the top of my list for that alone. But it is also loaded with vitamins as well. As much as I love to make tuna fish salad, that is NOT the way to go, because mayonnaise is made from RAW EGG WHITES which BLOCK the absorption of the B vitamins. Since we are eating the tuna for the B vitamins, slathering it in mayo is completely self-defeating. The best solution I have found is to make the tuna fish salad with regular yellow mustard instead of mayo. I sounds like it should taste awful, since the tuna has a very strong flavor and the mustard has an even stronger flavor, but it seems that the two cancel each other out. Give it a try, either I am right or my taste buds are ruined. I am not sure which it is!

OF PARTICULAR INTEREST

1) **NUTS and SEEDS** – Most nuts are loaded with vitamin E and minerals. Each nut usually has a high concentration of a specific mineral. Almonds are the highest in Vitamin E, pistachios are loaded with vitamin B6 and Brazil nuts are loaded with selenium (a rather hard to find trace mineral that we do need.) I try to include shelled nuts in my daily eating regimen in the form of a trail mix: 1) sunflower seeds (you know you can't go wrong there) 2) Raisins (aside from being sweet, these guys are very nutritious and loaded with iron) 3) almonds, 4) pistachios, 5) pumpkin seeds (high in zinc and magnesium) 6) walnuts, and 7) Brazil nuts. This is very nutritious but also the nuts bring a lot of calories with them, so we can't rely on them to meet our daily requirements of most of these essential nutrients unless we are also willing to burn off all of those extra calories that they bring.

2) **KIWIS, GUAVAS, ORANGES and GRAPEFRUIT** – Guavas are a bit more difficult to find in the produce section of most grocery stores but Kiwis have become a common mainstay in most grocery stores across the land and they are LOADED with vitamin C. Just two average sized kiwis will provide you with at least the average daily requirement of the GOOD NATURAL L-ascorbic acid form of vitamin C and this is HIGHLY PREFERRED over the manufactured form which is 50% of the BAD left-handed form of the molecule. (Actually the L means Left-handed! So the other stereoenantiomer that is created in the synthesis of the FAKE vitamin C is the WRONG WAY and TOXIC right-handed molecule.) One large orange or grapefruit will also take care of your Vitamin C for the day.

    END OF CHAPTER QUIZ

1. Which of the following is NOT a PRIMARY FOOD?
    A. Yogurt
    B. Turnip greens
    C. Cherries
    D. Corn
    Answer: D. Corn. This is a grain and is a SECONDARY FOOD which means it should be GREATLY REDUCED in

your daily eating regimen. The other three are excellent
healthy PRIMARY FOODS. PRIMARY FOODS should make
up the BULK of your daily eating regimen.
2. Which of the following are notable exceptions to the
SECONDARY FOOD types (are very healthy and can be eaten
regularly because of their health benefits):
    A. Wheat germ
    B. Oatmeal
    C. Chick peas
    D. All of the above.
    Answer: D. All of the above. Wheat germ is a grain product
    not included in the notable exceptions because it happens to
    be a SUPERFOOD! (An EXTREME EXCEPTION.)
3. Which of the following are loaded with essential nutrients rarely
found in any other food but they are potentially very FATTENING:
    A. Fruits
    B. Nuts
    C. Dairy products
    D. Both B and C
    Answer: D. Nuts are very densely packed with vitamin E and
    minerals that are usually difficult to find elsewhere and they
    are loaded with calories. Dairy products are also very healthy
    foods and are certainly fattening as well unless they are skim
    or lowfat versions.
4. Wheat germ is your best and most easily added to your daily
eating regimen source of:
    A. Zinc
    B. Magnesium
    C. Manganese
    D. Selenium
    Answer: C. Manganese. There are several excellent choices
    to choose from, but Wheat germ has some zinc and
    magnesium in it as well.
6. Sardines are a SUPERFOOD because they are loaded with;
    A. Zinc
    B. Vitamin B12
    C. DHA and EPA Moega-3 fatty acids
    D. Both B and C
    Answer: D. 3 to 5 ounces a day are excellent brain and heart
    food.
7. Which of the following is a superfood because it is loaded with
Zinc, Complete Protein, and several vitamins too?
    A. Pumpkin seeds
    B. Beef liver
    C. Lamb
    D. Tuna
    Answer: C. Lamb is one of the very best land animal foods on
    Earth.

Alright, so we know we need all 14 vitamins or 13 plus choline if you prefer. And we also need 14 minerals plus sulfur, some of them in trace quantities and some in shockingly large doses on a daily basis. If the vitamins are vital, the minerals are equally if not MORE IMPORTANT mainly because we rarely pay much attention to them and chronic deficiencies have been linked to everything terrible from diabetes to cancer to heart disease and heart attack. Cancer and heart failure together are responsible for the VAST MAJORITY of ALL DEATHS in the United States today numbering in the many HUNDREDS of THOUSANDS of victims each year and I believe that the VAST MAJORITY of all those tragic DEATHS ARE PREVENTABLE.

We also need no less than NINE essential amino acids in our diet as well. The good news is that they are all found in COMPLETE PROTEIN of "CP." The bad news for vegetarians, especially hard-core vegans is that NO PLANT has COMPLETE PROTEIN. They are ALL deficient in methionine and lysine and the methionine shortage is a REAL PROBLEM. (Although lysine deficiency is no walk in the park either.)

Then there are the Omega-3 fatty acids. While ALA is found in many plant foods, we cannot be completely sure that it is enough and the only source of DHA and EPA which are NECESSARY to brain and cardiovascular health is FISH. Even the most hard core vegans are going to have to rethink their belief system and start taking fish oil (which is a processed product of dubious quality) at the very least. There is little doubt that a purely vegetarian diet loaded with ALA will likely lead to reasonable healthy blood pressure and cholesterol levels but that does not change the fact that the HUMAN BODY MUST HAVE DHA and EPA and FISH (and other sea critters) are basically the ONLY SOURCE.

This, as a matter of fact, is exactly why the American public is being DECIMATED by heart disease and heart attacks because we normally do not eat much fish and THAT MUST CHANGE.

THE MINERAL AND ESSENTIAL NUTRIENTS LISTS

These are worth the cost of the book. I am going to lay out every nutrient (amino acids will just be called "CP" (COMPLETE PROTEIN which contains all of them) in at the very least the 100% RDA amounts and list every SUPERFOOD and its serving size that takes care of them: so no more guessing and no more confusion. You will have everything you need in a quick and easy to follow summary.

All we have to do then is list these and then list all of the foods that can cover them; then fill in the blanks each day and bingo you've got them all covered.

Personally I don't like to eat foods that have 20% of the daily requirement here and 30% there. I don't have time to mess around like that, patching together four and five different foods throughout the day just to make sure I have ONE nutrient covered. Multiply that by 41 and you will have a wall sized chart for every day of the week. That's about as useless as breasts on a bull, to coin a phrase, and it is equally UNNECESSARY.

KNOCKING MOST OUT WITH THE SUPERFOODS

Let's go down the list and see what can be taken care of quickly, easily, and conveniently with a single portion of the superfoods. NOTE: I cover the vitamins in Vol.2 – Vitamins.

THE MINERALS

If you have read carefully up to this point then you know that most people on Earth are suffering from chronic deficiencies not just of one mineral but likely MOST OF THEM and that is TERRIBLE for the body. I am amazed that I even survived to the age of thirty the way I was going. But it is never too late to fix the problem and get on track eating the proper foods. They can and will SAVE YOUR LIFE and make it longer, healthier, and happier too.

THE SUPERFOOD SHORT LIST FOR MINERALS

2 CUPS NATURAL ORGANIC YOGURT: >100% CALCIUM and IODINE.

5 oz. DARK CHOCOLATE (100% PURE CACAO): 100% IRON and MAGNESIUM, ≈50% COPPER

2 CUPS PUMPKIN SEEDS: 100% ZINC. Zinc is REAL TROUBLE. It is hard to find in sufficient quantities in our natural whole foods and is involved in upwards of a HUNDRED enzymatic processes involving virtually EVERY CELL in your body. Chronic deficiency can severely impede the immune system and make you susceptible to everything from the common cold to CANCER.

½ CUP SUNFLOWER SEED KERNELS: This is already on the menu resolving 100% RDA of B1, B5, and E as well as 76% of the B6. They also give you >100% PHOSPHORUS and SELENIUM, and ≈50% COPPER (They are the TOP SUPERFOOD on planet Earth. EAT THEM DAILY!)

1 oz. WHEAT GERM: >100% MANGANESE (rather than one slice of whole grain wheat bread and this superfood also provides 100% RDA of vitamins B7 and B9 as well.)

3 CUPS 100% CONCORD GRAPE JUICE: 100% CHROMIUM.

1 CUP COOKED OATMEAL: 100% MOLYBDENUM.

≈24 oz. LOW SODIUM VEGETABLE JUICE: 70% POTASSIUM.

1 tsp. IODIZED SALT: 100% SODIUM, CHLORINE and IODINE.

The ONLY mineral NOT on that list is SULFUR! ALL 14 ESSENTIAL MINERALS with known RDA's are COVERED by this list. 1 cup of BROCCOLI or 3 EGGS will load you up on SULFUR. But it is also in CP (COMPLETE PROTEIN) which is next.

THE NINE ESSENTIAL AMINO ACIDS (COMPLETE PROTEIN)

At least 110 grams (about 4 oz.) of CP are considered by the FDA to comprise the 100% RDA of CP (COMPLETE PROTEIN) which

contains all nine essential amino acids in reasonable quantities.
PLANT PROTEIN is deficient in TWO CRITICAL amino acids:
METHIONINE and LYSINE and you should NOT depend on plant
sources for your COMPLETE essential amino acid daily regimen.

THE SUPERFOODS LIST FOR CP

4 – 6 oz. BEEF, LAMB, TURKEY, CHICKEN, or FISH: >100% CP.
That's the entire list! Just eat animal meat and you are covered.

THE SUPERFOODS LIST FOR OMEGA-3 (DHA and EPA)

1Tbsp. COD LIVER OIL: >2600mg DHA/EPA.

1 oz. TUNA: ≈470mg DHA/EPA

1 oz. SARDINES: ≈360mg DHA/EPA

1 oz. ATLANTIC MACKEREL: ≈1,000mg DHA/EPA

1 oz. ALASKAN SALMON (wild-caught): ≈575mg DHA/EPA

DON'T FORGET YOUR VEGETABLE SOURCE OMEGA-3!

¼ CUP WALNUTS = 2,660mg ALA (alpha-linoleic acid)

The FDA is still trying to figure out the RDA for the Omega-3
fatty acids that are critical and often deficient essential nutrients in
the U.S. Since there are no known cases of overdosage toxicity, I
recommend setting that tablespoon of Cod Liver Oil as the
baseline for your daily uptake (2500+ milligrams daily for
EPA/DHA and a minimum of 1,500mg per day of ALA.)

END OF CHAPTER QUIZ

1. This superfood solves the RDA of calcium and iodine:
   A. 2 cups of natural organic yogurt
   B. 2 cups of pumpkin seeds
   C. 5 oz. dark chocolate
   D. 1 cup sunflower seed kernels
   Answer: A. 2 cups of natural organic yogurt cover our very
   high daily requirement of calcium and our trace requirement of
   iodine. The yogurt will also cover about ¼ of your Complete
   Protein requirement for the day as well.

2. This superfood solves the RDA of iron and magnesium:
   A. 2 cups of natural organic yogurt
   B. 2 cups of pumpkin seeds
   C. 5 oz. dark chocolate
   D. 1 cup sunflower seed kernels
   Answer: C. Just 5 oz. of PURE 100% CACAO will easily
   provide you with the rather high daily requirements of both
   iron and magnesium.

3. This superfood solves the RDA of zinc:
   A. 2 cups of natural organic yogurt
   B. 2 cups of pumpkin seeds
   C. 5 oz. dark chocolate
   D. 1 cup sunflower seed kernels
   Answer: B. 2 cups of pumpkin seeds are one of the few foods
   on planet Earth that can satisfy our high daily requirement of

zinc; a mineral that is HARD TO FIND in most of our foods in reasonable amounts.

4. This superfood solves the RDA of phosphorus and selenium:
    A. 2 cups of natural organic yogurt
    B. 2 cups of pumpkin seeds
    C. 5 oz. dark chocolate
    D. 1 cup sunflower seed kernels
    Answer: D. 1 cup of sunflower seed kernels each day will more than cover your needs for phosphorus and selenium which is HARD TO FIND in most foods.

5. The only people who are going to have a LOT of trouble getting all nine essential amino acids in their diet are:
    A. Americans because they prefer beef rather than fish
    B. People who only eat poultry
    C. People who only eat fish
    D. Strict vegetarians.
    Answer: D. All nine essential amino acids (essential means that you MUST get them in the foods you eat) are in CP (Complete Protein) which is found in animal whole meats of any kind and NOT plants.

6. The only people who are going to have an adequate supply of DHA/EPA Omega-3 fatty acids in their diet are:
    A. Americans because they prefer beef to fish
    B. People who only eat poultry
    C. People who only eat fish
    D. Strict vegetarians.
    Answer: C. FISH is the ONLY SOURCE on Earth of the GOOD forms of the Omega-3's that we MUST have in sufficient quantities on a daily basis.

7. This superfood source product can solve the DHA/EPA Omega-3 requirement easily:
    A. 2 cups of natural organic yogurt.
    B. 5oz. Dark chocolate
    C. 1 tablespoon of cod liver oil.
    D. None of the above.
    Answer: C. Just 1 Tbsp. of cod liver oil per day will provide you with ALL of the DHA/EPA Omega-3's the human body needs and brings a lot of animal source true vitamin A and D as well.:

8. Which of the following will help prevent diabetes?
    A. Eliminate "trash calories" like foods high in starch and processed cane sugar.
    B. 1 cup of broccoli slathered in a teaspoon of minced fresh garlic once a day
    C. 6 oz. sardines or tuna fish and 5 oz. 100% cacao daily,
    D. All of the above.
    Answer: D. All of the above. Ending a lifestyle loaded with high starch foods like potatoes and sugary sweets goes a long

way toward preventing diabetes. The broccoli and garlic is rich in chromium and the fish is rich in the important Omega-3's and Leucine while the dark chocolate is loaded with magnesium all of which help the body properly use and regulate blood sugar and can go a long way toward preventing late onset diabetes.

9. Which of the following can help prevent cancer?
A. Eliminating processed and packaged foods high in chemical additives.
B. Switching to all-natural whole foods diet
C. Getting ALL 41 essential nutrients in sufficient quantities in natural whole foods daily.
D. All of the above.
Answer: D. The only thing missing is exercise and you will be on the way to avoiding this dreadful disease. And don't forget that ALA, DHA, and EPA are the 3 vital Omega-3's that help to prevent cancer.

10. The ONE food loaded with molybdenum that is necessary for proper utilization of sulfur in our foods is:
A. Broccoli
B. Grape juice
C. Dark chocolate
D. Oatmeal
Answer: D. Oatmeal. This is the only readily available food that has MANY good nutrients for the body and is also packed with Molybdenum which allows us to metabolize sulfur.

11. The best source of manganese is:
A. Broccoli
B. Dark chocolate
C. Oatmeal
D. Wheat Germ
Answer: D. Wheat germ. Just ONE OUNCE has 100% RDA of manganese which shows up in many enzymes throughout the body.

12. Which superfood has Omega-3 and lots of vitamins as well?
A. Tuna
B. Sardines
C. Salmon
D. All of the above
Answer: D. All of the above. 10 oz. Tuna fish covers B3, B6 and D3 and about 5000mg of DHA/EPA. Just 3 oz. sardines cover B12 and about 1500mg of DHA/EPA. 7 oz. of Salmon covers B7 and D3 and choline and 3500mg of DHA/EPA.

THANK YOU AND GOD BLESS AND GOOD LUCK AND ABOVE ALL ELSE; TAKE CARE OF YOURSELF (BECAUSE NO ONE ELSE IS GOING TO DO IT!)

REFERENCES
Most information in this book was found at: wikipedia.org, nutritiondata.self.com, myfooddata.com, WebMD, draxe.com, whfoods.com, and the fda.gov and nih.gov. These websites are excellent resources and you should check them out.
[1] The data on about Calcium was found at:
* https://draxe.com/foods-high-in-calcium/ Retrieved on 07-30-2018
* https://www.myfooddata.com/articles/foods-high-in-calcium.php Retrieved on 07-30-2018
* http://www.whfoods.com/genpage.php?tname=nutrient&dbid=45 Retrieved on 07-30-2018

[2] The data about Iron was found at:
* https://draxe.com/top-10-iron-rich-foods/ Retrieved on 07-30-2018
* https://www.myfooddata.com/articles/food-sources-of-iron.php Retrieved on 07-30-2018
* http://www.whfoods.com/genpage.php?tname=nutrient&dbid=70 Retrieved on 07-30-2018

[3] The data about Phosphorus was found at:
* https://draxe.com/foods-high-in-phosphorus/ Retrieved on 07-30-2018
* https://www.myfooddata.com/articles/high-phosphorus-foods.php Retrieved on 07-30-2018
* http://www.whfoods.com/genpage.php?tname=nutrient&dbid= 127 Retrieved on 07-30-2018

[4] The data about Iodine was found at:
* https://draxe.com/iodine-rich-foods/ Retrieved on 07-26-2018
* https://www.myfooddata.com/articles/natural-foods-high-in-iodine.php Retrieved on 07-26-2018

[5] The data about Magnesium was found at:
* https://draxe.com/magnesium-deficient-top-10-magnesium-rich-foods-must-eating/ Retrieved on 07-30-2018
* https://www.myfooddata.com/articles/foods-high-in-magnesium.php Retrieved on 07-30-2018
* http://www.whfoods.com/genpage.php?tname=nutrient&dbid=75 Retrieved on 07-30-2018

[6] The data about Zinc was found at:
* https://draxe.com/foods-high-in-zinc/ Retrieved on 08-23-2018
* https://www.myfooddata.com/articles/high-zinc-foods.php Retrieved on 08-23-2018
* http://www.whfoods.com/genpage.php?tname=nutrient&dbid= 115 Retrieved on 08-23-2018

[7] The data about Selenium was found at:
* https://draxe.com/selenium-foods/ Retrieved on 08-23-2018
* https://www.myfooddata.com/articles/foods-high-in-selenium.php
Retrieved on 08-23-2018
* http://www.whfoods.com/genpage.php?tname=nutrient&dbid=95
Retrieved on 08-23-2018

[8] The data about Copper was found at:
* https://draxe.com/foods-high-in-copper/ Retrieved on 08-23-2018
* https://www.myfooddata.com/articles/high-copper-foods.php
Retrieved on 08-23-2018
* http://www.whfoods.com/genpage.php?tname=nutrient&dbid=53
Retrieved on 08-23-2018

[9] The data about Manganese was found at:
* https://draxe.com/manganese/ Retrieved on 08-23-2018
* https://www.myfooddata.com/articles/foods-high-in-
manganese.php Retrieved on 08-23-2018

[10] The data about Chromium was found at:
* https://draxe.com/what-is-chromium/ Retrieved on 08-23-2018
* http://www.whfoods.com/genpage.php?tname=nutrient&dbid=51
Retrieved on 08-23-2018

[11] The data about Molybdenum was found at:
* http://www.whfoods.com/genpage.php?tname=nutrient&dbid=
128 Retrieved on 08-29-2018

[12] The data about Potassium was found at:
* https://draxe.com/low-potassium/ Retrieved on 08-23-2018
* https://www.myfooddata.com/articles/food-sources-of-
potassium.php Retrieved on 08-23-2018

[13] The data about Sodium was found at:
* https://draxe.com/low-potassium/ Retrieved on 08-23-2018

[14] The data about the 9 Essential Amino Acids was found at:
* https://bareblends.com.au/blog/the-9-essential-amino-acids-
what-are-they-and-why-do-we-need-them/ Retrieved on 08-23-
2018

[15] The data about the Omega-3 Fatty Acids was found at:
* https://draxe.com/omega-3-benefits-plus-top-10-omega-3-foods-
list/ Retrieved on 08-23-2018
* https://www.myfooddata.com/articles/high-omega-3-foods.php
Retrieved on 08-23-2018